THE ERGOGENICS EDGE

Pushing the Limits of Sports Performance

MELVIN H. WILLIAMS, PhD
Old Dominion University

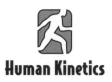

Human Kinetics

Dedicated to my fellow sport scientists throughout the world who study sport performance and the means to enhance it through safe, legal, and ethical means

Library of Congress Cataloging-in-Publication Data

Williams, Melvin H.
    The ergogenics edge : pushing the limits of sports performance /
Melvin H. Williams
      p.   cm.
    Includes bibliographical references and index.
    ISBN 0-88011-545-9
    1. Sports--Physiological aspects.   2. Doping in sports.   3. Energy
metabolism.   4. Dietary supplements.   I. Title.
RC1235.W55   1997
612'.044--dc21   97-19425
                                         CIP

ISBN: 0-88011-545-9

Developmental Editor: Kent Reel; **Assistant Editor:** Rebecca Crist; **Editorial Assistant:** Jennifer Hemphill; **Copyeditor:** Stephen Moore; **Proofreader:** Myla Smith; **Indexer:** Prottsman Indexing; **Graphic Designer:** Robert Reuther; **Graphic Artist:** Denise Lowry; **Photo Editor:** Boyd LaFoon; **Cover Designer:** Jack Davis; **Photographer (cover):** Claus Andersen; **Illustrator:** Doug Burnett and M.R. Greenberg; **Printer:** Versa Press

Human Kinetics books are available at special discounts for bulk purchase. Special editions or book excerpts can also be created to specification. For details, contact the Special Sales Manager at Human Kinetics.

Printed in the United States of America   10   9   8   7   6   5   4   3   2   1

Human Kinetics
Web site: http://www.humankinetics.com/

United States: Human Kinetics, P.O. Box 5076, Champaign, IL 61825-5076
1-800-747-4457
e-mail: humank@hkusa.com

Canada: Human Kinetics, Box 24040, Windsor, ON N8Y 4Y9
1-800-465-7301 (in Canada only)
e-mail: humank@hkcanada.com

Europe: Human Kinetics, P.O. Box IW14, Leeds LS16 6TR, United Kingdom
(44) 1132 781708
e-mail: humank@hkeurope.com

Australia: Human Kinetics, 57A Price Avenue, Lower Mitcham, South Australia 5062
(088) 277 1555
e-mail: humank@hkaustralia.com

New Zealand: Human Kinetics, P.O. Box 105-231, Auckland 1
(09) 523 3462
e-mail: humank@hknewz.com

CONTENTS

Preface v

Acknowledgments x

1 Factors Limiting Sports Performance . 1

2 Breaking Performance Barriers With Sports Ergogenics 9

3 Boosting Energy and Power 19

4 Building Mental Toughness 41

5 Getting a Mechanical Advantage . . . 59

6 Examining Performance Factors in Specific Sports 81

7 Answering Four Big Questions About Ergogenics 99

8 Rating the Sports Ergogenics 115

Appendix A 279

Appendix B 284

References 286

Index 308
About the Author 317

PREFACE

We all possess natural, innate athletic abilities. The nature of our athletic abilities depends to a great extent on the genes we have inherited from our parents; genes determine our height, our general body shape, our muscle fiber type, our ability to generate muscular energy, our psychological strength, and a multitude of other inborn characteristics that contribute to athletic success. Our genetic endowment helps determine what athletic achievements are possible. Every healthy athlete can sprint for 100 meters, but only a few can do it faster than 9.9 seconds.

Not all athletes have the genetic potential to be Olympic champions, but every athlete can achieve maximal genetic capacity through appropriate physiological, psychological, and biomechanical training. Over the past 40 years, exercise and sport scientists have conducted studies to help them understand the physiological, psychological, and biomechanical nature of athletic performance, often in attempts to help improve training programs and maximize human athletic potential. Athletes at all levels of competition have gone to extraordinary lengths in their specific sport training programs to help ensure victory against an opponent or to establish a new personal standard or record of performance. Adequate and proper training is the most effective means for an athlete to achieve specific sport performance goals.

Athletes at all levels of sports competition might wonder if special aids will help them improve performance above and beyond that attributable to training. Athletes search for substances or techniques that will provide them with an advantage (the so-called racer's edge) over their competitors, or the ability to exceed their own personal best or set records. Informal surveys with elite athletes reveal that before competition they are in such a psychological frame of mind that they will take anything to increase performance, provided it is not lethal. Athletes at lower levels of competition exhibit similar attitudes and behaviors, consuming a variety of nutritional compounds in the belief their performances will be enhanced.

Special substances or treatments used in attempts to improve physiological, psychological, or biomechanical functions important to sport are ergogenic aids, or *sports ergogenics;* ergogenic refers to an increase in the rate of work output.

I have had experience with sports ergogenics on several levels. As a college athlete I used nutritional sports ergogenics, such as protein supplements, in attempts to gain muscle mass for American football. As a marathoner and ultramarathoner I have used a legal pharmacological sports ergogenic, caffeine, in attempts to improve endurance. As a coach at both the high school and college levels I used psychological sports ergogenics in attempts to improve performance of my athletes (although I must admit that at the time I did not know them as psychological sports ergogenics). As a sport scientist the focus of my research for more than 30 years has been on sports ergogenics, including nutritional, pharmacological, psychological, and physiological sports ergogenics.

In 1983 I was fortunate to be in a position to edit the book *Ergogenic Aids in Sport* for Human Kinetics. Some of the leading sport scientists in the United States contributed to the book, which was developed primarily for our peers—other sport scientists. Later, Rainer Martens, the president of Human Kinetics, encouraged me to write *Beyond Training: How Athletes Enhance Performance Legally and Illegally,* a less technical book on ergogenic aids targeted not only at elite and college athletes and their coaches, but also at the recreational athlete who wants to do his or her best in sports competition, be it a local 10-kilometer road race, a minitriathlon, or any sport in which an athlete might benefit from the use of an appropriate ergogenic aid. *Beyond Training* was published in 1989, but considerable scientific research has been published since that time, and this book represents a significant revision and update.

Chapter 1 introduces the concept of sports performance factors (SPFs), and provides an overview of those inherited human attributes that determine the limits to sports performance and success.

Chapter 2 explores the ways different sports ergogenics might enhance specific SPFs.

Chapter 3 focuses on the development of physical power, or energy production, and provides an overview of how sports ergogenics may boost energy and power.

Chapter 4 centers on the development of mental strength, and includes a general discussion of psychological sports ergogenics as a means to increase mental toughness.

Chapter 5 concentrates on the use of physics to gain a mechanical edge in sport, including a general discussion on the application of biomechanical and mechanical sports ergogenics.

Chapter 6 helps you identify the SPFs that are important to your sport (see table 6.2) and provides a list of sports ergogenics (see table 6.3) that, theoretically, may enhance your specific SPFs.

Chapter 7 covers the importance of research in determining the effectiveness of alleged sports ergogenics, and highlights safety concerns, legal aspects, and ethical issues that may be associated with use of various sports ergogenics.

Chapter 8 is the heart of the book, providing information on the nature of each specific sports ergogenic, including the following points.

Classification and usage: What is it and how is it used?

Sports performance factors: Which athletes might benefit from its use?

Theory: How is it supposed to work?

Effectiveness: Does it work? Might it impair performance, that is, is it ergolytic, not ergogenic?

Safety: Are health risks associated with its use?

Legal aspects: Is its use legal in training or competition?

Ethical concerns: Are there any ethical issues associated with its use?

Recommendations: Are there sufficient grounds to recommend its use for training or sports competition?

Each sport has inherent, specific SPFs relative to physical power, mental strength, and mechanical edge. Some sports require high power, others low power. Athletes in some sports benefit from increased psychological arousal, others from relaxation. Athletes in some sports benefit greatly from improved mechanics, others less so. Sports ergogenics are designed to improve specific SPFs. Some are effective, others are not. Hundreds of sports ergogenics are marketed for use by athletes at all levels of sports competition. Unfortunately, claims regarding the effectiveness of many of these sport ergogenics are based on theoretical considerations, not on properly designed and conducted research.

This book is designed as a professional reference source to help you identify sports ergogenics that have been purported to enhance SPFs relative to your sport. You will find information on almost all alleged sports ergogenics, from A to Z, that have been studied over the past 20 years to determine their effectiveness, safety, legal status, and ethical concerns. Following an analysis of each of these points, a recommendation is provided.

One of the basic points underlying the recommendation of a specific sports ergogenic is its effectiveness, that is, does it do what it is theorized to do. Determination of the effectiveness of a sports ergogenic needs to be based on reputable research. I recommend no sports ergogenic unless research suggests it may be effective. Even if a sports ergogenic is effective, the general recommendation offered will be tempered by safety, legal, and ethical constraints. If a sports ergogenic poses a health risk, it cannot be recommended for use even though it may be a highly effective aid. Also, in my opinion, the use of any sports ergogenic considered to be illegal by various sports governing authorities, such as the International Olympic Committee, the National Collegiate Athletic Association, or the National Federation of High School Athletic Associations, should be considered unethical by the athlete. Thus, no prohibited sports ergogenic will be recommended for use, although it is recognized that this code of ethics is not universally supported by athletes.

Appendix A provides a list of common agents prohibited for use in sport. Not all drugs or techniques could be listed, but you may contact the United States Olympic Committee Drug Education Hotline, 800-233-0393, to obtain information on a specific drug. Be aware that all sport organizations have policies regarding the use of sports ergogenics, particularly drugs. Be familiar with the policies of your specific sport organization.

New dietary supplements marketed as sports ergogenics are introduced every year. Many contain individual ingredients or combinations of various substances discussed in this book. By checking the ingredients in the supplement, you may be able to evaluate its potential effectiveness by reading the appropriate section in this book. You can obtain additional information on alleged nutritional sports ergogenics by contacting the Gatorade Sport Science Institute, 800-616-4774, or the Food Nutrition Information Center at the National Agriculture Library, 301-504-5719, or the American College of Sports Medicine, 317-637-9200. These agencies may put you in contact with others who can provide you with information.

NOTICE

The purpose of this book is to serve as a reference source only. The information provided is designed to help athletes make informed decisions regarding the use of sports ergogenics as a means to enhance performance in sport. The effectiveness, safety concerns, legal status, and ethical issues of a specific sport ergogenic should be considered by all athletes prior to its use. No sport ergogenic that is deemed ineffective, unsafe, or illegal is recommended. The decision to use effective, safe, and legal sports ergogenics is left to the ethical judgment of the athlete.

ACKNOWLEDGMENTS

I would like to acknowledge deep gratitude to my many students and colleagues who have participated in our research efforts with ergogenic aids over the past 30 years, and to those sport scientists around the world who have conducted research in order to evaluate the effectiveness of numerous ergogenic aids. It is only through such well-controlled research that we may provide sound recommendations to those involved in sport regarding the use of purported sport ergogenics. Thanks to Sharon Jones, my research assistant, for her many hours in securing relevant research publications. Special thanks go to Rainer Martens for his incentive motivating me to develop several books on sport ergogenics for Human Kinetics, to Ted Miller for his encouragement and ideas in structuring this book, and to Kent Reel for his very cooperative and helpful support during the developmental and production processes. Sincere appreciation is extended to Stephen Moore, copyeditor, and Rebecca Crist, assistant editor, for a superb job; also to Denise Lowry and Robert Reuther, the graphic artists, and Boyd LaFoon, the photo editor, for the artwork to enhance the ideas presented in this book.

FACTORS LIMITING SPORTS PERFORMANCE

Play is basic to human nature. Children instinctively run, jump, and throw. To compete at play also is basic to human nature, and children become involved in elementary games, attempting to run faster, jump higher, or throw farther than their playmates.

As we age, we become involved in more sophisticated games, called *sports,* in which competition is a prime objective. The word *competition* is defined in a variety of ways. In relation to sport, competition is defined as a struggle for supremacy, a striving to do one's best or outperform one's competitors to win.

Society has valued sport supremacy since the origin of organized competition. Successful athletes, from the ancient Olympic Games to the contemporary sports scene, have reaped both fame and fortune. Today, star athletes appear on the covers of international magazines such as *Time* and *Newsweek;* Olympic heroes appear on cereal boxes; teenage athletes become instant multimillionaires.

Because of the many benefits associated with sport success, athletes are always trying to improve their performances, usually under the guidance of skilled trainers (coaches). Whereas in the past trainers relied primarily on experience and observation to help improve sports performance, today, though observation and experience are still important, trainers of elite athletes also have access to a team of sport scientists. These specialists may provide physiological, psychological, and biomechanical analyses to help improve sports performance.

SPORTS PERFORMANCE IMPROVEMENT

With few exceptions, the improvement in sports performance and the resultant breaking of established records has continued unabated for 100 years. Not long ago the 4-minute mile, the 7-foot high jump, and the 15-foot pole vault were considered ultimate sport performances. More recently, athletes have surpassed the 3:45 mile (see figure 1.1), the 8-foot high jump, and the 20-foot pole vault. Similar accomplishments

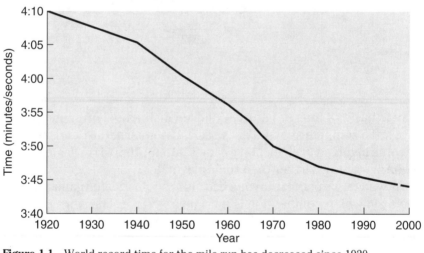

Figure 1.1 World record time for the mile run has decreased since 1920.

have been made in a variety of sports at national and international levels of competition as well as those in high schools and colleges. High school athletes are performing better in some sports than Olympic champions did 30 years ago.

The Olympic motto is *citius, altius, fortius*, translated as "swifter, higher, stronger."

Sport achievement continues to improve for many reasons. Larger population and greater opportunities for sports participation increase the genetic pool of potential record breakers. Better coaching and training methods improve the athlete's physiological fitness level, psychological strategies, and biomechanical technique. Better nutrition and medical treatment help the athlete train more effectively. Technological improvements in facilities and equipment design provide mechanical or biomechanical advantages. Individually and collectively, these are the major reasons sports records are broken.

LIMITS TO SPORTS PERFORMANCE

Are there limits to sports performance? If so, what are they? I believe the ultimate barrier is the inability to achieve optimal production, control, and efficient use of energy, for energy is the basis of all movement in sport.

Two factors play significant roles in energy production and utilization in sport: *genetic endowment* and *training*. Heredity provides us with certain physical abilities to produce energy, but to succeed in sport we have to maximize or control our ability to produce energy and use it as efficiently as possible. Even if we are born with the characteristics of a natural athlete, we must train hard to realize our potential.

The innate ability of Lance Armstrong, one of America's elite cyclists, was demonstrated at age 15 when his aerobic capacity placed him in the upper 1 to 2 percent of athletes worldwide.

— *Jay Kearney, senior sports physiologist, USOC*

Intervention into genetic potential to enhance sports performance has not been applied extensively. The human genome project (an international research project designed to determine the functions of all human genes) is nearly complete, however, so identification of genes responsible for the expression of physiological, psychological, and biomechanical characteristics essential to sports success might make such intervention possible, and even probable.

On the other hand, the application of science to sports training has mushroomed in the past 30 years. *Sport physiologists* have studied different training methods and nutritional practices to improve performance; *sport psychologists* have used psychological approaches to remove mental barriers to performance; and motor learning specialists and *sport biomechanists* have investigated ways to learn and execute specific sport skills. Much of this research has focused on ways to lower barriers to human performance.

Three general types of barriers to optimal performance in sport that can be controlled to some degree are physiological, psychological, and biomechanical barriers. *Physiological barriers* limit the ability to produce energy. *Psychological barriers* limit the ability to control energy. *Biomechanical barriers* limit the ability to use energy efficiently. The three barriers may be interrelated. For example, a psychological barrier to performance might interfere with optimal production of energy by physiological processes and might disrupt optimal biomechanical utilization of energy.

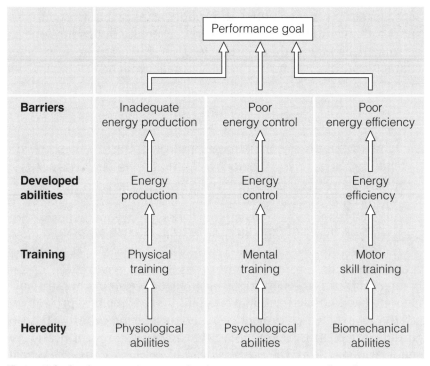

Figure 1.2 Inadequate energy production, poor energy control, and poor energy efficiency are barriers to achieving performance goals.

An extended discussion of the production, utilization, and control of energy and associated fatigue processes appears in subsequent chapters. At this point it is sufficient to note general physiological, psychological, and biomechanical limitations to human performance. Figure 1.2 highlights some of these barriers.

Although you cannot modify your genetic potential (you did not get a chance to choose your parents), you can maximize what sports potential you do have through training. You might not have the natural athletic ability of another, but proper training can develop your inherited abilities to the level necessary for you to achieve your goal. Proper training is the most effective means you have for improving your sports performance.

> **T**o become an Olympic athlete, choose your parents well.
>
> *— Per-Olaf Åstrand, world-famous physiologist*

SPORT SUCCESS AND SPORT TRAINING

Sport success is in the eye of the beholder. Consider athletes running a 26.2-mile (42.2-kilometer) marathon. Success for one athlete might be completing a full marathon, a worthy goal in itself. For another athlete, success might mean winning an age-group award in a local marathon. For yet another athlete, success might be winning the gold medal in the Olympic marathon or being the first to cross the finish line in Boston. Similar comparisons can be made for other sports from youth through international competitions (figure 1.3).

To be all that you can be in sport, you need to optimize your sport training. Whether you are attempting to complete your first marathon or to win the Olympic gold, the sport training principles are the same. At the United States Olympic Training Center, the sports training program attempts to overcome physiological, psychological, and biomechanical barriers by focusing on three aspects of sport performance: physical power, mental strength, and mechanical edge. *Physical power* represents energy production, *mental strength* involves energy control, and *mechanical edge* relates to energy efficiency.

Each sport makes different demands on energy production, control, and efficiency; these demands are referred to as *sports performance factors.*

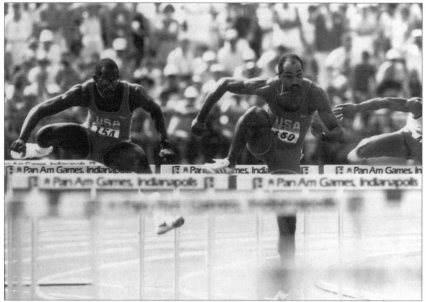

© Claus Andersen

Figure 1.3 To be Olympic class an athlete must inherit specific sport abilities, and must maximize these abilities through intense training.

SPORTS PERFORMANCE FACTORS (SPFs)

Hundreds of different sports competitions are held around the world. There were 271 finals in the 1996 Olympic Games, not including the numerous finals in the subsequent Paralympics for athletes with impaired mobility and vision. Each sport event, from archery to yachting, requires that participants possess certain abilities to be successful. We shall refer to these abilities as *sports performance factors (SPFs)*.

Scientists have analyzed a variety of sports events from a physiological, psychological, and biomechanical perspective to determine the SPFs critical for successful performance. Genetics and training are key determinants of SPFs in an athlete. Genetics plays a key but variable role in all SPFs. Although some SPFs, such as body height, might not be modifiable, scientists note that most SPFs, such as muscular strength, can be improved significantly through proper training aimed at achieving one's genetic potential.

Scientists have classified SPFs by using a number of approaches, some more detailed than others. For example, muscular strength may be labeled simply as strength, or in such specific subdivisions as static strength, dynamic strength, explosive strength, upper-body strength, and lower-body strength. Dozens of basic SPFs have been identified, but I have compressed them into three general categories: (a) physical power, (b) mental strength, and (c) mechanical edge, with several subdivisions as highlighted in table 1.1. An expanded discussion of the relationship of SPFs to the three general categories is presented in chapters 3, 4, and 5.

TABLE 1.1
Sports Performance Factors

Physical power (energy production)
Explosive power and strength
High power and speed
Power endurance
Aerobic power
Aerobic endurance

Mental strength (neuromuscular control)
Stimulation
Relaxation

Mechanical edge (efficiency)
Increase muscle/body mass
Decrease body fat/body mass

As mentioned, proper training is the most effective way for an athlete to improve sports performance. Training can increase physical power and mental strength, and provide a mechanical edge. Athletes, however, may seek methods they feel might substitute for training or go beyond training to increase their physical power, mental strength, or mechanical edge; in such cases they turn to sports performance aids, or sports ergogenics.

BREAKING PERFORMANCE BARRIERS WITH SPORTS ERGOGENICS

Scientific literature refers to substances that athletes use to help enhance performance as ergogenic aids, or *sports ergogenics*. The term *ergogenic* is derived from the Greek words *ergon* (work) and *gennan* (to produce). Hence, an ergogenic usually refers to something that produces or enhances work. Business and industry managers have extensively applied the science of *ergonomics* to increase work output. These ergonomic developments range from designing computers for increased secretarial comfort and work productivity to using complex robots for assembling automobiles. In this sense we all use some form of ergogenics to make work easier in our daily tasks or to increase productivity.

From the earliest days of organized sports competition, athletes have used sports ergogenics in attempts to improve athletic performance beyond what would be possible through natural ability (genetics) and training alone. In ancient Greece and Rome, athletes focused on nutritional aids. They may have believed, for example, that specific body organs of animals contained certain attributes, such as the courage of the lion in its heart, which could be transferred to the athletes if they ate the organ. More than 100 years ago, however, numerous athletes—including boxers, marathon runners, baseball and soccer players, European cyclists, Olympians, and others—experimented instead with using such drugs as alcohol, caffeine, and cocaine in attempts to improve their athletic abilities. In recent years phenomenal increases in sports science research, specifically in the areas of sports nutrition, sports psychology, sports biomechanics, and even sports pharmacology, have paralleled the development of virtually hundreds of purported sports ergogenics aimed at lowering barriers to human athletic performance.

The purpose of most sports ergogenics is to improve performance by enhancing physical power (energy production), mental strength (energy control), or mechanical edge (energy efficiency), thus preventing or delaying the onset of fatigue. Table 2.1 highlights the

---

TABLE 2.1
Enhancing Sports Performance Through Physical Power, Mental Strength, and Mechanical Edge

To enhance physical power
1. Increase the amount of muscle tissue used to generate energy.
2. Increase the rate of metabolic processes that generate energy within the muscle.
3. Increase the energy supply in the muscle for greater duration.
4. Improve the delivery of energy supplies to the muscle.
5. Counteract the accumulation of substances in the body that interfere with optimal energy production.

To enhance mental strength
1. Increase psychological processes that maximize energy production.
2. Decrease factors that interfere with optimal psychological functioning.

To enhance mechanical edge
1. Improve human body biomechanics to increase efficiency by decreasing body mass, primarily body fat.
2. Improve human body biomechanics to increase stability by increasing body mass, primarily muscle mass.

specific methods whereby sports ergogenics could enhance sports performance.

Athletes might use sports ergogenics in any one of the three major areas listed in table 2.1, usually for a specific purpose. They could take carbohydrate supplements to enhance physical power by increasing the energy supply in the muscle; they could try hypnosis to enhance mental strength by eliminating negative thoughts; they could don aerodynamic racing suits to enhance the mechanical edge by decreasing air resistance. Some sports ergogenics can elicit multiple effects. For example, anabolic or androgenic steroids can enhance physical power by increasing muscle mass, mental strength by increasing aggressiveness, and mechanical edge by increasing overall body weight, all of which might improve performance in a specific sport, such as sumo wrestling.

CLASSIFICATION OF SPORTS ERGOGENICS

Sports ergogenics can be classified in a variety of ways. In *Beyond Training: How Athletes Enhance Performance Legally and Illegally,* I listed five categories: (a) nutritional aids, (b) pharmacological aids, (c) physiological aids, (d) psychological aids, and (e) mechanical or biomechanical aids.

Some sport ergogenics are actually training techniques: for example, psychological sports ergogenics, such as imagery or transcendental meditation. As with physical training, athletes must practice specific psychological skills in order to enhance mental strength. Mechanical and biomechanical sports ergogenics represent a form of training as well. Biomechanical skill improvement through the use of mechanical aids, such as a hand paddle in swimming, requires dedicated training to improve energy efficiency. Additionally, sport clothing and sport equipment are designed to provide a mechanical edge, but the athlete must train with them to maximize the potential benefits. Nevertheless, because psychological skill training, biomechanical skill training, and clothing and equipment can also be regarded as sports ergogenics that might help improve sports performance, I have presented an expanded discussion of them in chapters 3 and 4.

For my purposes in this book, I will consider as sports ergogenics only substances that are taken into the body (or related techniques to increase the intake of such substances) in attempts to increase physical power, enhance mental strength, or provide a mechanical edge, primarily by acting favorably on one or more of the processes listed in table 2.1. These substances may be grouped into three classes of sports ergogenics—nutritional, pharmacological, and physiological.

Nutritional Sports Ergogenics

Nutritional sports ergogenics primarily serve to increase muscle tissue, muscle energy supplies, and the rate of energy production in the muscle. Although most nutritional sports ergogenics are designed to increase physical power, some also may contribute to mental strength or mechanical edge.

The foods you eat can provide more than 50 nutrients, all essential to energy production in one way or another. You would be amazed at the variety of functions these essential nutrients perform in order to help control energy production in your body. In essence, however, these nutrients act on three basic functions relative to energy processes: (a) some nutrients serve as an energy source; (b) some regulate the processes whereby energy is produced in the body; and (c) some provide for growth, development, and structure of the various body tissues that produce energy (see figure 2.1).

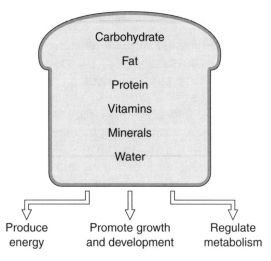

Figure 2.1 The nutrients that you eat serve three basic functions in your body.

Proper nutrition is essential for optimal sports performance. If you are deficient in a nutrient that is important to energy production during exercise, your performance will suffer. Generally speaking, if you eat a varied diet containing wholesome foods, you are not likely to suffer from a nutrient deficiency that will impair sports performance.

You can obtain all the nutrients you need for optimal sports performance from a well-balanced diet. The nutrients you eat may be grouped into six different classes: carbohydrates, fats, proteins, vitamins, minerals, and water. In general, carbohydrates serve as a source of energy. Fats provide energy, too, but they are also part of the structure of most cells. Protein plays a variety of roles, being necessary for (a) tissue formation, growth, and development; (b) enzyme formation to regulate energy production; and (c) energy, as a source under certain conditions. Vitamins primarily regulate a variety of metabolic processes by working with enzymes. Many minerals also are involved in the regulation of metabolism, but some contribute to the structure of your body as well. Finally, water comprises most of your body weight and helps to regulate a variety of body processes. Table 2.2 presents the nutrients currently believed to be essential for life.

All nutrients are involved in energy production in one way or another, but some specific nutrients are especially important to the athlete whose rate of energy production may be increased tremendously during exercise. For example, protein is the foundation for forming muscle tissue, carbohydrates are a prime energy source in the muscle, and iron is essential for transporting adequate oxygen to the muscle cell.

Table 2.3 highlights those nutrients that have been studied in relation to sports performance; you'll find further discussion of them in chapter 8.

Pharmacological Sports Ergogenics

Pharmacological sports ergogenics are drugs designed to function like hormones or neurotransmitter substances that are found naturally in the human body. Like some nutritional sports ergogenics, pharmacological sports ergogenics may enhance physical power by affecting various metabolic processes associated with sport success. For example, amphetamines may mimic the effects of epinephrine (adrenaline), a hormone secreted naturally during exercise that enhances physiological processes involved in energy production. Pharmacological sports ergogenics also may affect mental strength and mechanical edge.

Pharmacological sports ergogenics have raised the most concern among athletic governing bodies. *Doping,* or the use of drugs by athletes in attempts to improve performance, has persisted for nearly

TABLE 2.2
Essential Nutrients for Humans

Carbohydrates
   Fiber

Fats (essential fatty acids)
   Linoleic fatty acid   Alpha-linolenic fatty acid

Proteins (essential amino acids)

Histidine	Phenylalanine
Isoleucine	Threonine
Leucine	Tryptophan
Lysine	Valine
Methionine	

Vitamins

Water-soluble	*Fat soluble*
Thiamine (B_1)	A (retinol)
Riboflavin (B_2)	D (calciferol)
Niacin	E (alpha-tocopherol)
Pyridoxine (B_6)	K (phylloquinone)
Pantothenic acid	
Folic acid	
B_{12}	
Biotin	
Ascorbic acid (C)	

Minerals

Major	*Trace*	
Calcium	Chromium	Molybdenum
Chloride	Cobalt	Nickel
Magnesium	Copper	Selenium
Phosphorus	Fluorine	Silicon
Potassium	Iodine	Tin
Sodium	Iron	Vanadium
Sulfur	Manganese	Zinc

Water

TABLE 2.3
Nutritional Sports Ergogenics

Carbohydrate

Carbohydrate supplements

Fats

Fat supplements

Omega-3 fatty acids

Medium-chain triglycerides

Protein/amino acids

Protein supplements

Branched-chain amino acids (BCAA)

Arginine, lysine, ornithine

Tryptophan

Aspartates

Vitamins

Antioxidants

Pantothenic acid

Thiamine (B_1)

Folic acid

Riboflavin (B_2)

B_{12}

Niacin

Ascorbic acid (C)

Pyridoxine (B_6)

Vitamin E

Minerals

Boron

Phosphates

Calcium

Selenium

Chromium

Vanadium

Iron

Zinc

Magnesium

Water

Fluid supplements

Plant extracts

Anabolic phytosterols

Yohimbine

Ginseng

Miscellaneous

Bee pollen

Engineered dietary supplements

HMB (beta-hydroxy-beta-methylbutyrate)

Multivitamins/minerals

Vitamin B_{15}

a century, but it was only after World War II that doping became rampant among athletes involved in international competition and professional sports. Doping eventually filtered down to college sports, and today appears to pervade sports even at the high school and middle school levels.

A 14-year-old South African runner recently tested positive for anabolic steroids, the youngest track and field athlete ever accused of using pharmacological sports ergogenics.

Although some drugs may be effective sports ergogenics, their use might also significantly increase health risks. The Medical Commission of the International Olympic Committee (IOC) notes that doping

---

TABLE 2.4
Major Pharmacological Substances and Methods
Prohibited by the International Olympic Committee (IOC)
With Some Examples

Prohibited substances
Stimulants (amphetamine, cocaine, ephedrine)
Narcotics (narcotic analgesics)
Anabolics (anabolic steroids, clenbuterol)
Diuretics
Peptide and glycoprotein hormones and analogues

Prohibited methods
Blood doping
Pharmacological, chemical, and physical manipulation

Classes of drugs subject to certain restrictions
Alcohol
Caffeine
Marijuana
Local anesthetics
Corticosteroids
Beta-blockers
Specified beta-2 agonists (Clenbuterol)

violates the ethics of both sport and medical science and is prohibited. Most athletic governing bodies, such as the IOC, the United States Olympic Committee (USOC), the National Collegiate Athletic Association (NCAA), the National Football League (NFL), and the National Basketball Association (NBA) have developed drug-use policies. Any athlete competing under the jurisdiction of a specific athletic governing body should be aware of its drug rules and regulations.

Most organizations pattern their rules after the IOC, which bans those major classes of drugs and methods listed in table 2.4. Most of the substances and methods are covered in chapter 8, and an expanded list is presented in appendix A.

Physiological Sports Ergogenics

Physiological sports ergogenics are substances or techniques designed specifically to augment natural physiological processes that generate physical power. Examples include blood doping, erythropoietin, and oxygen inhalation. Physiological sports ergogenics are not drugs per se. In a strict sense, however, some may be regarded as drugs because they are proscribed substances. Several have been prohibited by the IOC, so we might refer to them as *physiological doping agents,* or *nonpharmacological doping.*

Other physiological sports ergogenics may be related to nutritional sports ergogenics. Carnitine and creatine are found in foods we eat,

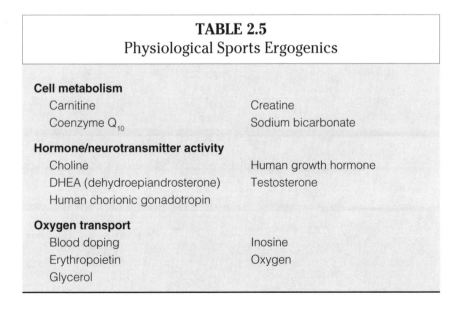

TABLE 2.5
Physiological Sports Ergogenics

Cell metabolism

Carnitine	Creatine
Coenzyme Q_{10}	Sodium bicarbonate

Hormone/neurotransmitter activity

Choline	Human growth hormone
DHEA (dehydroepiandrosterone)	Testosterone
Human chorionic gonadotropin	

Oxygen transport

Blood doping	Inosine
Erythropoietin	Oxygen
Glycerol	

but they are nonessential nutrients because they are formed in the body from other nutrients. In general, these nonessential nutrients are intimately involved in specific physiological processes important to sports performance.

Table 2.5 highlights those physiological sports ergogenics that have been studied in relation to sport performance. (See also chapter 8.)

In the next three chapters we shall expand our discussion of physical power, mental strength, and mechanical edge, and provide some general indications of how nutritional, pharmacological, and physiological sports ergogenics may be used in attempts to enhance specific sports performance factors.

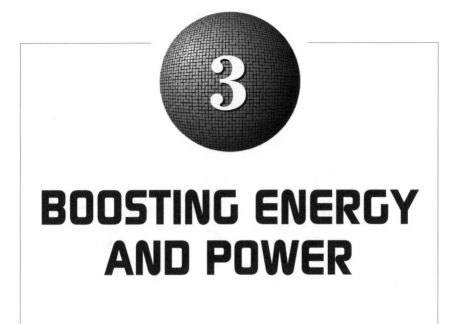

BOOSTING ENERGY AND POWER

Sport involves energy, which exists in six forms in nature (see table 3.1). A key principle of energy is that one form can be converted into another. Nuclear energy released from uranium in a nuclear power plant undergoes various conversions before generating light in a lamp. Scientists have learned to control much of the energy in nature to help make our lives easier and more comfortable. Your body also can convert one form of energy into another, and sport scientists are investigating the optimal application of energy principles to human physical performance.

TABLE 3.1
Forms of Energy in Nature

Form of Energy	Example
Light	Light from the sun
Nuclear	Fission from uranium
Electrical	Electricity from lightning
Chemical	Carbohydrates in food
Thermal	Body heat produced in exercise
Mechanical	Movement such as lifting weights

SPORT ENERGY

Two principal forms of energy that are important to sport are *mechanical energy* and *chemical energy*. Sport involves movement, which is mechanical energy. Chemical energy is stored in our bodies in a variety of forms and is used to produce movement.

Electrochemical energy and *heat energy* also play important roles in sport performance. Electrochemical energy produced by our nervous systems is needed to release chemical energy in our muscles, providing energy for muscle contraction and resultant movement. Just as a telephone system uses electricity to allow us to communicate with one another, the nervous system uses electricity, in the form of ions, to allow our brains to communicate with our muscles. Any disruption in the production or proper application of this electrochemical energy in the body could lead to suboptimal performance. Heat energy is generated continuously in our bodies when chemical stores are used, but may increase markedly during exercise. Excess accumulation or loss of body heat during exercise can impair performance.

PHYSICAL POWER AND ENERGY PRODUCTION

In order to understand how to enhance your sport performance, you need to understand how the human body stores and uses energy, and the possible causes of impairment, such as fatigue or inefficient utilization.

Optimal sport performance depends upon optimal energy production (physical power), control (mental strength), and efficiency (mechanical edge). We will elaborate on the last two principles in chapters 4 and 5. For now, though, let's illustrate the principle of physical power by drawing an analogy between your body and an automobile.

Optimizing physical power production in sports requires the right engine to produce energy. To compete in the Indianapolis 500, you need a racing machine; your family sedan simply will not cut it. As an analogy, your muscles are your engines. They must be capable of processing your chemical energy sources at a rate optimal for specific sports. For some sports you need powerful engines that produce energy rapidly for short periods of time; for others you need smaller, more efficient engines that produce energy for prolonged periods. You also must have enough of the right type of chemical energy, or fuel, stored in your body. Most cars function properly on ordinary un-leaded gasoline, some need premium grades, while high-speed compe-tition race cars require special mixtures for optimal performance. Like a car, your body runs on fuel. The type of fuel your body uses depends

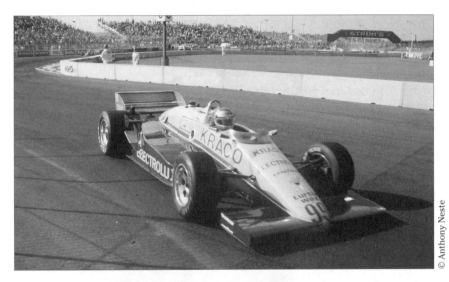

© Anthony Neste

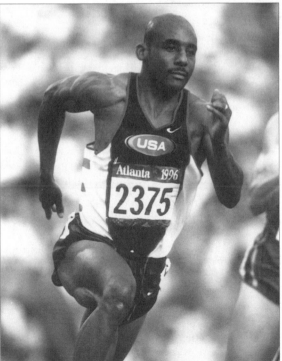

© Claus Andersen

Figure 3.1 The sophis-ticated racing car must have a powerful engine; the world-class sprinter needs powerful muscles, the engines of human movement.

on the energy demands of a given sport. You have two general types of muscle engines that are designed to store and use several different types of chemical energy, or fuel. Some are designed for high power output (figure 3.1), others for endurance.

Energy production is the basis of physical power, and the muscle fiber type is the basis of energy production. It is the engine of sport.

Muscle Fiber Types

Muscles provide the means for human movement by contracting (shortening) and moving the bones to which they are attached. Figure 3.2 is an illustration of a muscle connected to a bone via its tendon.

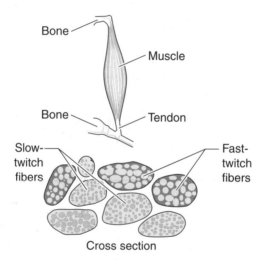

Figure 3.2 The muscle contains thousands of individual muscle cells, some fast-twitch, some slow-twitch.

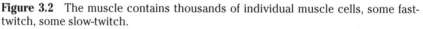

Each whole muscle contains varying numbers of *motor units,* and each motor unit is composed of varying numbers of individual *muscle cells* or *fibers.* A key point is that muscle fibers come in different types, based primarily on the contraction speed (although all fibers in each motor unit are of the same type). A single contraction of a fiber is a *twitch.* In general, some muscle fibers shorten at a high rate of speed and are known as *fast-twitch (FT) muscle fibers;* others shorten at a slower rate and are known as *slow-twitch (ST) muscle fibers.*

Energy Systems and ATP

The rate at which a muscle fiber contracts depends on its ability to convert its chemical energy into mechanical energy, the latter being the actual shortening of the muscle cell. Your muscles contain three distinct systems that determine the rate of energy production for movement. One is called the *ATP-CP energy system,* the second is the *lactic acid energy system,* and the third is the *oxygen energy system.* Each muscle fiber possesses all three energy systems, but the dominance of one system over another determines the primary energy characteristics of the individual muscle fiber.

Although your muscles possess three different energy systems, only one form of energy is utilized to cause the muscle to contract. This form is ATP, the abbreviation for *adenosine triphosphate,* a high-energy chemical compound found in all muscle cells. Stimulation of a muscle by a nerve impulse results in a series of electrochemical events, leading to the breakdown of ATP, the release of chemical energy, and the harnessing of this energy for muscle contraction (see figure 3.3). ATP is the immediate and essential source of energy for muscle contraction. Without it, your muscle cannot contract. The muscle contains only a very small amount of ATP, about enough for you to expend energy at your maximal rate for only 1 second. Additional ATP must be supplied if muscle contraction is to continue. The faster you want your muscles to contract, the more rapidly you must replenish ATP. The purpose of the three energy systems is to supply this additional ATP, but the rate at which they can supply it varies.

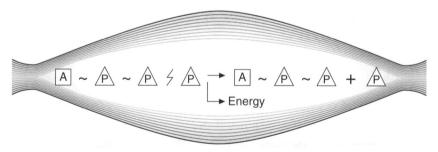

Figure 3.3 Adenosine triphosphate (ATP) is the immediate source of energy for muscle contraction. When the end phosphate is split off, energy is released.

ATP-CP Energy System

The ATP-CP energy system consists of ATP and another high-energy phosphate compound, CP *(creatine phosphate).* ATP is the immediate source of energy for muscle contraction. It can release energy very rapidly, but as noted, it is in very limited supply. CP also may break down and release energy very rapidly, but this energy cannot be used directly for muscle contraction. Instead, its role is to resynthesize ATP rapidly (see figure 3.4). CP supply also is limited in the muscle, however, and may be able to resynthesize ATP for only an additional 5 to 10 seconds or so. Although all muscles contain the ATP-CP energy system, the ability to use ATP and CP rapidly is a primary characteristic of the FT muscle fibers. This energy system does not need oxygen (is not *aerobic*) in order to perform, and thus is an *anaerobic* (without oxygen) source of energy. The ATP-CP energy system is capable of producing energy very rapidly for short periods of time.

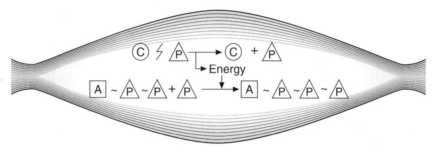

Figure 3.4 Creatine phosphate splits to release energy for the rapid resynthesis of ATP.

Lactic Acid Energy System

The lactic acid energy system uses carbohydrate as fuel, primarily in the form of glycogen stored in the muscles. The breakdown of *muscle glycogen* is known as *glycogenolysis.* This leads to a process called *glycolysis,* in which ATP can be produced rapidly, although not as rapidly as in the breakdown of CP.

Glycolysis may occur both in the presence and absence of oxygen. Under normal resting conditions your muscles' ATP requirement is relatively low, so glycolysis proceeds at a slower rate and can be sustained by the oxygen you take in. This aerobic energy production from carbohydrate accounts for about 40 percent of your energy demands at rest. As you begin to exercise, the rate of aerobic glycolysis increases to help meet your need for additional ATP.

Glycolysis that occurs without oxygen also contributes to energy production. As you increase your exercise intensity you eventually will reach a point at which your aerobic glycolysis cannot support energy production, primarily because you cannot take in and deliver enough oxygen to your muscle cells. Proportionately more of the ATP is now produced without adequate oxygen, through *anaerobic glyco-*

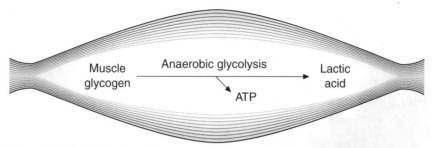

Figure 3.5 In the lactic acid energy system, muscle glycogen (carbohydrate) can break down to form ATP in the absence of adequate oxygen, but lactic acid is formed.

lysis (see figure 3.5). Through a series of chemical reactions in the muscle cell, the formation of lactic acid allows anaerobic glycolysis to continue. The accumulation of excess lactic acid, however, has been associated with fatigue processes within the muscle cell, limiting its effectiveness during exercise. The lactic acid energy system, therefore, is capable of producing energy at a fairly rapid rate, but it cannot produce energy for prolonged periods.

Oxygen Energy System

The oxygen energy system uses a variety of fuels to produce ATP, but depends primarily on *carbohydrates* and *fats*. The main source of carbohydrate for muscular energy during exercise is glucose that, as noted, is stored in limited supplies in the muscle as glycogen. Additional glucose is stored in the liver as glycogen and is released into the blood for delivery to the muscle when needed, although the supply in the liver is even more limited than that in the muscles. The main source of fat for muscular energy during exercise is *free fatty acids (FFA)*. Some fats, known as *triglycerides,* are stored in limited supply in the muscle and break down into FFA for entry into the oxygen energy system. Much of the fat in our bodies, however, is stored just under the skin and in some deeper areas, and these sources can provide substantial amounts of FFA. *Protein* normally is not used for energy production to any great extent, but under some conditions may become a significant source of energy for the oxygen energy system.

The oxygen energy system, as its name implies, needs an adequate supply of oxygen delivered to the muscles to help release the chemical energy stored in carbohydrates and fats. In contrast to the two anaerobic energy systems, the oxygen energy system is *aerobic*. Figure 3.6 provides a graphic overview of the oxygen energy system and its fuel sources.

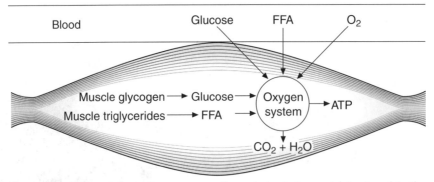

Figure 3.6 The oxygen system uses mostly carbohydrates and fats stored in the muscle or delivered by the blood as fuels.

Although the oxygen system cannot produce ATP as rapidly as can the two anaerobic systems, it can produce much greater quantities of ATP at a somewhat slower rate. Moreover, the rate at which the oxygen energy system produces ATP is dependent upon the type of fuel. For a given amount of oxygen, you may release more energy for exercise if you use carbohydrate instead of fat. In other words, carbohydrate is a more efficient fuel than fat. Unfortunately, the ability to store carbohydrate in the muscles and liver is limited for certain prolonged endurance events, whereas the body's fat supplies are extensive. Thus, while the oxygen energy system is designed for endurance, an insufficient supply of the optimal fuel, carbohydrate, can limit performance. Let us briefly explore the use of carbohydrate and fat as fuels for exercise.

Carbohydrate Use During Exercise. Almost all carbohydrate in your diet is broken down by the digestive process and liver into glucose, appearing as blood glucose or blood sugar. Some carbohydrate foods, particularly those rich in simple carbohydrates, have a high *glycemic index,* that is, they rapidly increase blood sugar. Other carbohydrate foods, such as fiber-rich legumes and vegetables, have a low glycemic index.

An increased blood glucose level stimulates the release of the hormone *insulin* from your pancreas. Insulin facilitates the transport of glucose from the blood into tissues in the body, most notably the liver and the muscles, where it is converted to its storage form, glycogen. If you eat more carbohydrates than you need, they will be stored as fat. These processes are depicted in figure 3.7.

Muscle glycogen regenerates ATP, enabling muscle contraction to

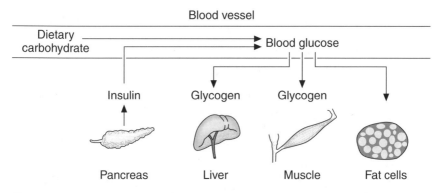

Figure 3.7 Dietary carbohydrate is converted into blood glucose. High blood glucose levels stimulate the pancreas to release insulin, which helps transport glucose into the muscles and other tissues. For athletes, adequate stores of muscle glycogen, liver glycogen, and blood glucose are important.

continue. As noted, muscle glycogen is the fuel in the FT muscle fibers for the lactic acid energy system, which predominates in intense, prolonged anaerobic exercise tasks. Glycogen in the ST muscle fiber is the preferred fuel for the oxygen energy system during high-level aerobic exercise.

The rate at which you use muscle glycogen stores depends primarily upon how intensely you exercise. If you perform high-speed anaerobic exercise, you use the glycogen in your FT fibers at a fast rate. This type of exercise may result in the rapid production of lactic acid, leading to the early development of fatigue.

During aerobic exercise you use a combination of muscle glycogen and fats as the energy sources in your ST muscle fibers. As you increase the intensity of your aerobic exercise, however, you use proportionally more glycogen than fats because glycogen is a more efficient fuel. In essence, you obtain about 7 percent more energy when you use glycogen instead of fats. Depending on how well trained you are, you may be able to use the muscle glycogen in your ST muscle fibers and exercise at a high percentage of your maximal oxygen uptake without accumulating excess lactic acid, and thus may continue to exercise for a prolonged period of time.

You normally cannot store large amounts of glycogen in your muscles, so glycogen may last for only an hour or so of high-level aerobic exercise. As your muscle glycogen stores deplete during prolonged exercise, your blood helps deliver glucose from the liver to your muscles, allowing you to maintain energy production at a given level. Because liver glycogen stores also are limited, however, they eventually will be unable to provide adequate glucose to the blood.

As discussed in chapter 8, carbohydrate supplementation may be an effective nutritional sports ergogenic.

Fat Use During Exercise. Following digestion and processing by the liver, dietary triglycerides are stored in your body, primarily as muscle triglycerides and *adipose* (fat) cell triglycerides. Dietary fats play a number of different metabolic roles in the body, one of the most significant of which is to serve as a fuel for the oxygen energy system. Fat, however, is a less efficient fuel than carbohydrate; fat produces less ATP per liter of oxygen consumed and produces it at a slower rate. Total energy demand is not great during rest and low-intensity exercise, so fat may provide 50 to 70 percent or more of the energy needs. As exercise intensity increases, the muscles begin to use increasing amounts of carbohydrate and proportionally lesser amounts of fat.

Figure 3.8 presents a schematic of fat as an energy source during exercise. Fat is stored as triglycerides in both muscle and adipose tissue. During exercise the muscle triglycerides break down into free fatty acids (FFA) and glycerol, and the FFA eventually is processed into the *mitochondria* (energy-producing factories in the cells) to provide ATP via the oxygen energy system. Glycerol is released into the blood

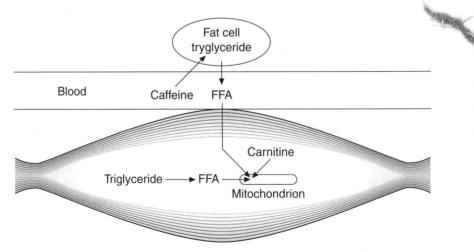

Figure 3.8 Fat can be used as an energy source during exercise. Triglycerides in fat cells release free fatty acids (FFA) into the blood for transport to the muscle. Supplies in the muscle also may be used. Fat supplementation, caffeine, and carnitine are several sports ergogenics used in attempts to improve the use of fats during exercise.

for transport to the liver for further metabolism. The adipose tissue throughout the body, under the influence of hormones such as epinephrine (adrenaline), also breaks down its triglycerides, with the FFA traveling via the blood to the muscles and the glycerol going to the liver.

As you become better trained aerobically, your muscles make several adaptations to help improve your performance. In essence, they develop a greater ability to use both carbohydrates and fats as sources of energy during exercise. The ability to oxidize fats at a faster rate allows you to substitute fat for carbohydrate as an energy source at a given speed. By using proportionately more fat, exercise training helps you spare some of your carbohydrate stores.

As discussed in chapter 8, various dietary strategies for increasing the use of fat as an energy source during prolonged aerobic endurance exercise have been used in attempts to enhance performance.

Supply and Support of the Energy Systems

Although the ability of the three energy systems to produce energy for movement resides in the muscle cell itself, each system needs a proper supply and support system in order to function at optimal capacity.

The ATP-CP system, as noted, uses ATP as the immediate source of energy for muscular contraction, and all three systems are designed to replace ATP. Thus, CP must be replenished in order for this energy system to operate. Energy released from the breakdown of ATP is used to resynthesize CP. The ATP used to resynthesize CP, however, ultimately is derived from the oxygen energy system. This process occurs during the recovery period between contractions.

The lactic acid energy system operates primarily in the FT muscle fibers and uses muscle glycogen, or carbohydrate, as its source of energy. Carbohydrate must be replenished in the FT fibers in order for this energy system to function adequately. Moreover, the accumulation of lactic acid in the muscle cell has been identified as a factor in the development of fatigue, so it must be removed rapidly.

The oxygen energy system operates primarily in the ST muscle fibers. To function properly, it needs an adequate supply of oxygen as well as replenishment of the proper fuel, either muscle glycogen or free fatty acids (FFA).

Each of the three energy systems needs an adequate supply of vitamins, minerals, and other substances in order to function effectively. The B vitamins are essential for processing carbohydrate for energy, minerals such as calcium are critical for regulating muscle contraction, and vitamin-like substances such as carnitine help process fat for energy. Because one of the byproducts of energy production for movement in the body is heat, the body must be able to dissipate this excess heat in order to function at an optimal level. In this regard, water is an essential nutrient for athletes who exercise under warm or hot environmental conditions.

The *cardiovascular system,* consisting of the heart and blood vessels, is the primary support system because it transports blood to and from the muscle cell. As the blood flows through the body it picks up oxygen from the respiratory system in the lungs; glucose from the liver; FFA from fat (adipose) tissue; a variety of nutrients including vitamins, minerals, and water from the digestive system; and hormones, such as adrenaline, from the endocrine system for delivery to the muscle cells in support of energy production. The blood also removes byproducts of energy metabolism, such as lactic acid and excess heat, that can interfere with optimal energy production within the muscle cell (see figure 3.9).

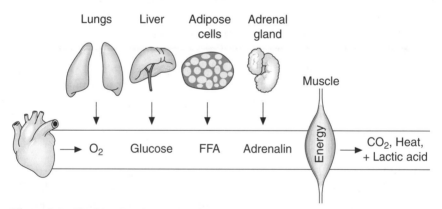

Figure 3.9 The blood is the main supply system to the muscles during exercise. It picks up and delivers oxygen, nutrients, and hormones from other tissues and removes byproducts of energy metabolism.

Optimal sport performance thus requires not only proper development of the appropriate energy system within the muscle cells, but also well-developed supply and support systems. Improvement in the supply and support systems may lead to improved energy production within the muscle cells.

Rates of Energy Production and Muscle Fiber Type

The rate of energy production depends primarily on two factors: (a) the muscle fiber type, and (b) the type of fuel that is used within the muscle.

Energy Production and Muscle Fiber Type

As noted, the body has several different muscle fiber types, classified for our purposes as fast-twitch (FT) and slow-twitch (ST) fibers. Both types of muscle fibers use ATP as the immediate source of energy for muscle contraction, but they replenish ATP at different rates. Both muscle fiber types use all three human energy systems to produce energy, but the FT muscle fibers use primarily the ATP-CP and lactic acid energy systems, whereas the ST fibers use primarily the oxygen system. As noted, the oxygen system cannot replenish ATP as rapidly as can the other two systems.

Success in specific types of sport or athletic endeavors appears to be related to the muscle fiber types you possess. Let us look briefly at the rates of energy production and their relationships to sport performance, using several events in elite male track athletics as a basis for comparison. In some events, such as the 100-meter dash, athletes need to produce energy very rapidly for a very short period of time, say 10 seconds or less. In this case, a high percentage of energy is derived from the ATP-CP system, so athletes with greater proportions of FT muscle fibers and highly developed ATP-CP systems may have the greater potential for success.

The sprint start may depend primarily on ATP, but subsequent speed depends on CP. In a world-class 400-meter dash (0.25 mile), energy must be generated rapidly for a longer period of time, less than 45 seconds. In such an event, the lactic acid energy system will provide most of the energy, so athletes with high capacities for anaerobic glycolysis might be more successful. In longer distances, such as 10,000 meters (6.2 miles) run under 27 minutes, energy is provided primarily by the oxygen energy system with carbohydrate as the major fuel. Those with high aerobic capacities, therefore, are more likely to be successful.

Energy Production and Types of Physical Power

In almost all types of sport events, with the possible exception of very brief maximal efforts, all three energy systems are used to one degree or another. ATP is always used, and it is replaced from CP, anaerobic glycolysis, and aerobic glycolysis dependent on the exercise intensity. In general, no single energy system is used exclusively, but there is a blending and overlapping of the energy derived from each energy system in the range from rest to explosive power. The rate at which energy is generated by the muscle is *power,* and the time that a certain level of power continues to be generated is *endurance.* We will subdivide the three energy systems into five types of power and endurance, as described below.

Explosive Strength and Power (ATP-CP Energy System).   Strength represents the neuromuscular ability to exert force and involves static or isometric strength, such as that required during a stalemate in arm wrestling, or dynamic or isotonic strength, such as that used for lifting a barbell. *Explosive strength,* often referred to as power or explosive power, is the ability to use dynamic strength very rapidly (in a second or so), such as in a sprint start in a 100-meter dash. ATP is the primary energy source used to generate explosive power (figure 3.10).

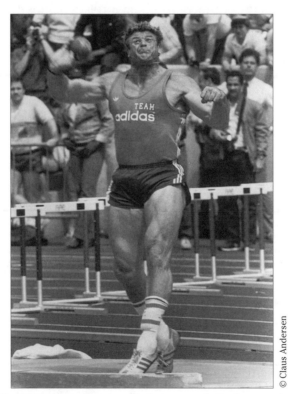

© Claus Andersen

Figure 3.10   Explosive strength, or explosive power, is the key sport performance factor in a maximum power effort.

The cheetah can accelerate from 0 to 70 miles per hour in 3 seconds.

High Power and Speed (ATP-CP Energy System).   Speed, or high power, represents the ability to develop muscular force rapidly for somewhat longer periods of time (5–30 seconds) compared to explosive power. Speed is anaerobic power. In track, 100- to 200-meter dash performance depends on speed. High levels of static strength may need to be maintained for similar time frames. CP is the primary energy source used to generate speed and high levels of static strength.

Power Endurance (Lactic Acid Energy System).   Power endurance, or anaerobic endurance, is the ability to sustain high levels of muscle force development for 1–2 minutes, such as when running a 400- or 800-meter race (see figure 3.11). In sports such as soccer, prolonged

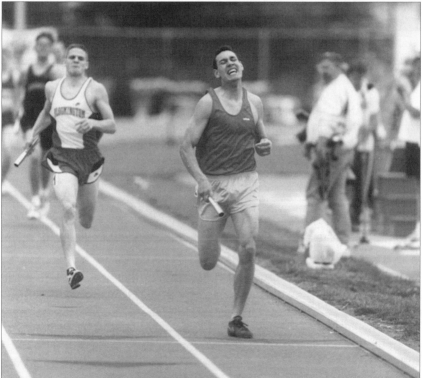

© Human Kinetics/Tom Roberts

Figure 3.11   In the finish of a 400-meter or 800-meter race, lactic acid accumulation elicits pain sensations as expressed on the faces of these runners.

intermittent high power leads to progressive increases in lactic acid and thus may be considered a form of power endurance. Muscle glycogen is the primary energy source used by the FT muscle fiber to generate power endurance.

Aerobic Power (Oxygen Energy System).   Aerobic power represents the ability to utilize oxygen at a high percentage of maximal. Such events may last 13–30 minutes or so. Running events such as 5–10 kilometers (3.1–6.2 miles) require aerobic power. Muscle glycogen is the primary energy source used by the ST muscle fiber, and some FT muscle fibers, to generate aerobic power.

The pronghorn deer of the North American prairies can cruise at 35 miles per hour for miles.

Aerobic Endurance (Oxygen Energy System).   Aerobic endurance is the ability to use oxygen at somewhat lower rates than aerobic power, but for prolonged periods such as 2 hours or more. Running events such as marathons and ultramarathons require aerobic endurance. Muscle glycogen, liver glycogen, muscle triglycerides, and plasma free fatty acids are the primary fuels used to generate aerobic endurance.

Table 3.2 summarizes the characteristics of each of the three energy systems, and their corresponding relationships to the various forms of physical power, found in the muscle cells.

PHYSICAL POWER TRAINING

Scientific evidence suggests that each of us is born with a specific distribution of muscle fiber types—that is, some of us may have a greater proportion of ST muscle fibers, while others may have more FT muscle fibers. In general, the distribution of muscle fiber types in men and women is similar, and untrained individuals possess about 50 percent of each type, although there is a wide range of distribution. Research has shown that elite sprinters have a greater proportion of FT fibers, and thus can generate explosive power and speed. Conversely, elite distance runners have more ST fibers, and thus are better able to develop aerobic power and endurance. Even though these elite athletes may have inherited specific muscle fiber types conducive to sport success, they must train intensely to maximize their elite potential.

TABLE 3.2

Major Characteristics of Muscle Energy Systems

	ATP-CP	ATP-CP	LACTIC ACID	OXYGEN	OXYGEN
Predominant muscle fiber type	FT	FT	FT	ST	ST
Main energy source	ATP	CP	Muscle glycogen	Muscle glycogen	Muscle glycogen and triglycerides; free fatty acids
Exercise intensity	Highest	Higher	High	Lower	Lowest
Rate of ATP use/ production	Highest	Higher	High	Lower	Lowest
Power production	Highest	Higher	High	Lower	Lowest
Capacity for total ATP production	Lowest	Lower	Low	Higher	Highest
Endurance	Lowest	Lower	Low	Higher	Highest
Oxygen needed	No	No	No	Yes	Yes
Anaerobic/ aerobic	Anaerobic	Anaerobic	Anaerobic	Aerobic	Aerobic
Typical track or running event	Sprint start	100-meter dash	800-meter run	2-km to 10-km run	Marathon and ultra-marathon
Time factor at maximal use	0-1 second	1-10 seconds	40-120 seconds	5-30 minutes	2 hours or more
Sports performance factor (SPF)	Explosive power	High power	Power endurance	Aerobic power	Aerobic endurance

You can't be a champion in a week or a year. You must accept a time of suffering.

— *Hassiba Boulmerka, women's Olympic champion, 1500 meters*

The amount of each type of muscle fiber you possess may have important implications for sport. Even if you haven't inherited the potential to perform at the elite level, however, you can maximize the capacity of each of your three energy systems through proper training. A properly balanced training program for a distance runner, for example, will improve the ability of both fiber types to use the oxygen energy system, thus improving the ability to produce energy more rapidly without fatigue over long distances.

The development of physical power is dependent on several major training principles. A number of excellent books are available for those who desire more details on the application of these principles to specific sports. Table 3.3 highlights the major training principles for physical power.

TABLE 3.3
Training Principles for Physical Power

Overload principle

The specific energy system used to generate physical power must be stressed beyond normal levels of activity. The energy system may be stressed in three ways: (a) increased exercise intensity; (b) increased exercise duration; (c) increased exercise frequency. For example, to increase strength you need to overload your muscles by some type of resistance strength-training program.

Progression principle

The overload on the specific energy system must be increased progressively as the muscle continues to adapt to training. For example, as you get stronger with resistance strength training, you may increase the amount of weights lifted during training.

Specificity principle

The overload and progression must be targeted to a specific energy system within a specific muscle group. Metabolic specificity refers to training a specific energy system, whereas neuromuscular specificity refers to training specific muscle groups. To develop strength in the thigh muscles, for example, you must overload the ATP-CP energy system in those muscles.

Reversibility principle

The overload, progression, and specificity principles must be applied continuously. For example, strength gains will be lost if resistance strength training is discontinued.

Although proper training will enhance your sport performance, your performance will be limited by your ability to generate ATP to sustain a given level of energy expenditure. When you exceed this capacity, fatigue sets in.

PHYSICAL POWER AND FATIGUE

An athlete who could run the 100-meter dash in 10 seconds would be able to run the marathon in 1:10:20, nearly an hour faster than the current world record, if the average pace for the 100-meter dash could be maintained. Such an attempt would be foolhardy, for the energy systems in the human body are not equipped to sustain such a pace. An athlete making such an attempt would slow down before completing 400 meters because of premature fatigue.

Fatigue is the enemy of almost all athletes; premature development of fatigue leads to a decrease in athletic performance (see figure 3.12). Fatigue is a complex phenomenon; it takes a variety of forms and has a number of definitions. For purposes of this book, *fatigue* is the inability to utilize your human energy resources to their fullest potential.

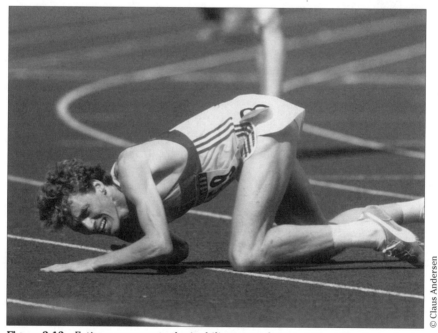

© Claus Andersen

Figure 3.12 Fatigue represents the inability to produce energy at the desired rate.

Fatigue may be caused by inadequate physical power, such as an inadequate energy supply in the muscles or an inability to produce energy fast enough. Fatigue can be caused by insufficient mental strength, such as the psychological inability to concentrate on the task at hand or improper execution of a sport skill due to mental interference from overstimulation. Fatigue also can be caused by a deficient mechanical edge, such as an inefficient body composition consisting of too much body fat. We will discuss psychological and biomechanical causes of fatigue in chapters 4 and 5, but the following discussion highlights the major factors underlying fatigue of physical power production.

Figure 3.13 represents some of the possible fatigue sites in the human body. The following discussion is keyed to the numbers in the figure.

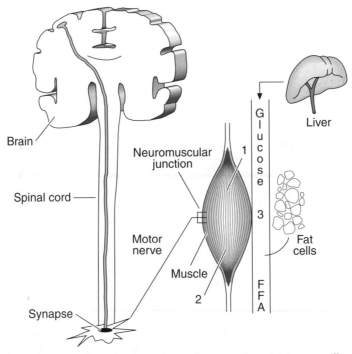

Figure 3.13 Possible fatigue sites exist in the muscular system, as well as in the cardiovascular system (see text).

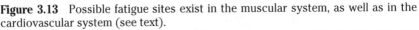

1. The muscle cell may contain inadequate amounts of energy stores, such as creatine as CP or carbohydrate in the form of glycogen. Creatine is essential for the ATP-CP energy system, and muscle glycogen is the essential fuel source for the lactic acid energy system and is the most efficient fuel for the oxygen energy system.

2. Another fatigue site could result from the inability of the electrical impulse to initiate the contraction process in the muscle. It has been theorized, for example, that excess acidity in the muscle cell due to lactic acid accumulation blocks some of the key steps in the processes that initiate muscle contraction.

3. The blood supply to the muscle may be a significant contributing factor to the development of fatigue. An inadequate delivery of nutrients such as glucose and FFA, low oxygen levels, and impaired ability to remove lactic acid or heat may adversely affect the performance of both the muscular system and the nervous system during exercise.

As mentioned, proper training is the most effective way for an athlete to delay fatigue and improve sports performance. Training can increase physical power and mental strength, and provide a mechanical edge. Athletes might seek methods to substitute for or to go beyond training in efforts to increase their physical power, mental strength, or competitive edge; in such cases they turn to sports ergogenics.

SPORTS ERGOGENICS FOR PHYSICAL POWER

The optimal production and utilization of muscle power is a key factor in sport success. Power production is dependent on (a) the size and type of muscle tissue, (b) the amount and type of fuel in the muscle, (c) the efficiency of the muscle metabolic pathways to process the fuel, (d) an efficient support system to supply the muscle with appropriate substances (such as fuel and oxygen), and (e) a support system to remove metabolic waste products.

Table 3.4 lists five ways that sports ergogenics may be used in attempts to increase physical power, and provides an example of specific nutritional, pharmacological, and physiological sports ergogenics that have been studied to determine their efficacy to induce such effects.

Chapter 6 lists nutritional, pharmacological, and physiological sports ergogenics that are purported to increase physical power sports performance factors (SPFs), specifically explosive power, high power, power endurance, aerobic power, and aerobic endurance. Chapter 8 provides details relative to the effectiveness, safety, legal status, and ethics of these purported sports ergogenics.

TABLE 3.4
Use of Sports Ergogenics to Increase Physical Power

1. Increase the amount of muscle tissue used to generate energy
   Nutritional ergogenics: Amino acids
   Pharmacologic ergogenics: Anabolic steroids
   Physiologic ergogenics: Human growth hormone
2. Increase the rate of metabolic processes that generate energy within the muscle
   Nutritional ergogenics: Vitamins
   Pharmacologic ergogenics: Stimulants
   Physiologic ergogenics: Carnitine
3. Increase the energy supply in the muscle for greater duration
   Nutritional ergogenics: Carbohydrate
   Pharmacologic ergogenics: Alcohol
   Physiologic ergogenics: Creatine
4. Improve the delivery of energy supplies to the muscle
   Nutritional ergogenics: Iron
   Pharmacologic ergogenics: Caffeine
   Physiologic ergogenics: Blood doping
5. Counteract the accumulation of substances in the body that interfere with optimal energy production (lactate, free radicals)
   Nutritional ergogenics: Antioxidant vitamins
   Pharmacologic ergogenics: Anti-inflammatory agents
   Physiologic ergogenics: Sodium bicarbonate

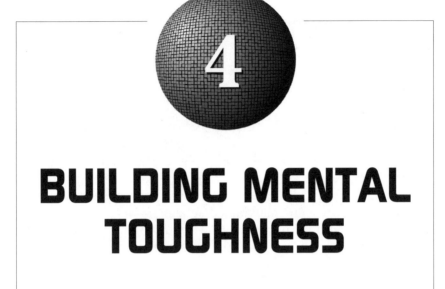

BUILDING MENTAL TOUGHNESS

If you want to optimize sport performance, you must control the production of energy by your muscles and the application of energy to movement.

In chapter 3 we compared your body to a car in terms of energy production. As does an automobile engine, your body needs the right engine (your muscles) to generate the desired power output. A high-tech racing automobile has a sophisticated computer system designed to control most functions of the car, including fuel injection and steering, to help maximize speed and rapidly influence the automobile's direction. In a similar fashion, your nervous system acts like a computer in your body. It controls the rate of energy production in your muscles to control their speed, and activates those muscles needed to move your body.

In chapter 3 we introduced the basic principles of training for physical power. Later in this chapter we discuss the general concept of mental training. Here we will discuss a basic principle of training relevant to the role of the nervous system in sport performance. This is the principle of *specificity,* of which there are two types: *neuromuscular specificity* (use of proper muscle groups) and *metabolic specificity* (rate of energy expenditure). Proper training of sport performance factors (SPFs) enables your nervous system to do two things: Call into play the proper muscle groups, and control the rate at which those muscles expend energy.

THE NERVOUS SYSTEM AND CONTROL OF MUSCLE FUNCTION

You probably are aware that the nervous system controls most of your body functions, including movement. *Nerve cells,* or *neurons,* create electrical impulses that are transmitted throughout your body. Neural stimulation of a particular body tissue initiates a response that is characteristic of that tissue. For example, neural stimulation of your adrenal gland releases adrenaline into your blood, whereas stimulation of your muscle cell causes it to contract and cause movement.

Figure 4.1 represents a simplified schematic of a *neural pathway* between the brain and a muscle cell. An electrical impulse is generated by a specific neuron in an area of the brain that controls the muscles. This impulse then passes along the neuron down to your spinal cord, where it communicates with another neuron. An electrical impulse

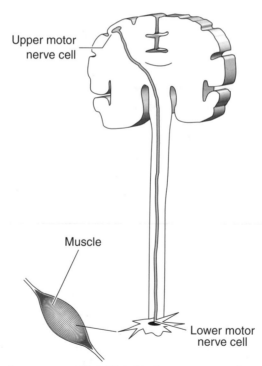

Figure 4.1 Voluntary movement is initiated in the motor control center in the brain. The simple pathway illustrated here represents a direct pathway between the brain and the motor nerve cell in the spinal cord.

generated in this neuron enables your spinal cord to communicate with specific muscle fibers and initiates a muscle contraction.

Unfortunately the control of human movement, particularly the complex movement patterns found in most sports, is not that simple. The central nervous system, including many parts of the brain and the spinal cord, functions much like a high-speed computer. It receives input, analyzes this input, and generates output.

During most sports activity the *central nervous system (CNS)* receives a variety of information (input) from various receptors in our bodies, including our eyes, inner ears, muscles, and joints. The central nervous system rapidly processes this information and initiates impulses to the necessary muscles for the desired movement patterns (output). Figure 4.2 illustrates some of the neural control mechanisms for human movement. (Be aware that this illustration is a gross oversimplification.)

Think about the first time you tried a complex sport skill, such as serving a tennis ball, swimming the front crawl, or skiing parallel turns. Do you remember how hard you had to concentrate in order to

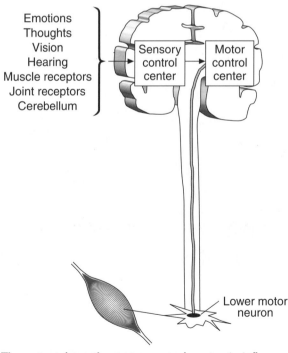

Figure 4.2 The output from the motor control center is influenced by various sensory control centers in different parts of the brain.

perform the skill properly? As you practiced, however, the skill became almost second nature and required less concentration. One theory of learning suggests that, as you learn to perform a complex sport skill, your central nervous system (hardware) develops a kind of computerized program (software) for that skill, and a given stimulus triggers a set pattern of muscular responses. For example, after you have perfected your tennis serve, throwing the ball into the air might initiate a programmed sequence in your nervous system that eventually results in the proper sequence and timing of muscle contractions and a smooth movement pattern (see figure 4.3).

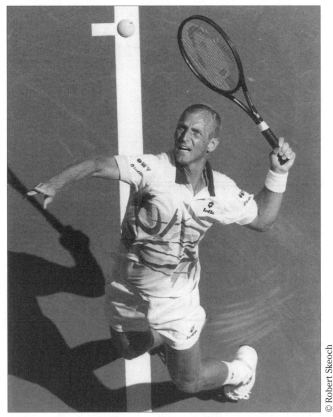

© Robert Skeoch

Figure 4.3 Many sports involve complex neuromuscular skills that need to be developed through proper training.

To attain optimal efficiency in sports it is critical that we learn and perfect the most effective techniques or skills for enhancing success. Another goal for athletes training in complex sports skills is to reach the point at which the skill becomes second nature, so that the athlete can concentrate on other aspects of the competition.

The nervous system plays an essential role as the control center for human movement. When you learn to do a sport skill efficiently, through proper coaching and much practice, your nervous system develops a programmed sequence of muscular contractions that allow you to perform the skill at maximal efficiency and effectiveness, enabling you to apply your energy most productively during competition. This process is referred to as *neuromuscular specificity of training* because we train the specific muscles involved in complex movements in any given sport. In other words, the best way to become more efficient in bicycling is to use those muscles involved in cycling. Cycling muscles are best developed through bicycling training, not through swimming or running training.

THE NERVOUS SYSTEM AND CONTROL OF ENERGY

The nervous system not only controls the muscles that are activated to do a particular sport skill, but also controls the amount of energy released in these muscles and how fast this energy is released. The nerve cells in your central nervous system serve specific muscle cells. Some go to the fast-twitch (FT) muscle fibers; others go to the slow-twitch (ST) fibers. Activation of these fibers causes either a fast or slow muscle contraction. The nervous system controls the amount of energy developed in several other ways. It may activate more muscle fibers, or it may activate them more frequently. A nerve fiber that goes to 50 ST muscle fibers and fires at a rate of 10 impulses per second will not generate nearly as much force as a nerve fiber going to 200 FT muscle fibers and firing at a rate of 50 per second. Because the nervous system controls this process, the muscles are in essence the slaves of the nervous system.

The nervous system also is important for the control of energy production because it helps to control the supply and support system to the muscle cells. For example, the nervous system helps channel the delivery of more blood to the muscles active during exercise, such as to your thigh muscles during bicycling, by helping open the blood vessels to those muscles. The nervous system also stimulates certain glands in the body to secrete hormones in the blood, which may then facilitate fuel supply to and energy production in the muscle cells. One key hormone discussed later is epinephrine (adrenaline); athletes have taken similar compounds in attempts to improve performance.

In essence, the nervous system controls the three energy systems within the muscle cells and hence the generation of physical power. To improve physical power, you must train the specific energy system or systems that are needed for a given SPF. This is referred to as *metabolic specificity of training.* In other words, you need to train at an intensity level comparable to that experienced in competition. If you are training for a 400-meter dash, you must occasionally train at speeds that will stress the lactic acid energy system. You must train your nervous system to activate your FT fibers more effectively, for they use the lactic acid energy system. As you continue to train, your body will make specific beneficial adjustments in the energy systems within the muscle cells and in the energy support systems, leading to an increased ability to produce energy during exercise.

MENTAL STRENGTH FROM STIMULATION TO RELAXATION

Mental strength represents the ability of the nervous system, particularly the conscious brain, to optimize energy production in the muscle and to control muscle movements. As we have seen, the nervous system controls not only the specific muscles, but also how fast and how powerfully they contract.

When we train properly, the nervous system and the muscles begin to function more efficiently. We develop neuromuscular skills, referred to as *perceptual-motor skills.* Perceptual-motor skills involve three basic components: (a) perception by the peripheral nervous system of a stimulus, which can be a stimulus from the muscle itself (such as a change in length) or a stimulus from the environment (such as visual input of a tennis ball); (b) interpretation of this stimulus by the CNS, primarily the brain; and (c) the motor response, or activation of specific muscles, in response to the stimulus.

We possess many perceptual-motor skills, and depending on the sport, some are more important than others. The four perceptual-motor skills presented in table 4.1 are relevant to specific types of sport performance.

Although perceptual-motor skills are controlled by specific areas in the brain and spinal cord, this control can be affected by parts of the

---

TABLE 4.1
Perceptual-Motor Abilities

Reaction time. Reaction time is the time elapsed between stimulation and the initial reaction to that stimulation. The stimulus may be visual (a tennis ball coming at you), auditory (the sound of the ball off your opponent's racket), or tactile (the impact of the ball on your racket).

Visual skills. Visual skills other than reaction time are important for some sports. Tracking is the ability to follow moving objects with both eyes, and is important in sports like tennis. Other factors such as peripheral vision and color sensitivity may be important for specific sports. For example, in Olympic archery events, competitors who are better able to perceive the color red may have an advantage.

Fine motor control. Fine motor control is precise neuromuscular regulation of muscle activity required in sports demanding precision and accuracy, such as archery and pistol shooting.

Gross motor control. Gross motor control is precise neuromuscular regulation of muscle activity required in sports demanding total body movement, such as during a rally in tennis. Coordination, agility, and balance are common terms associated with gross motor control.

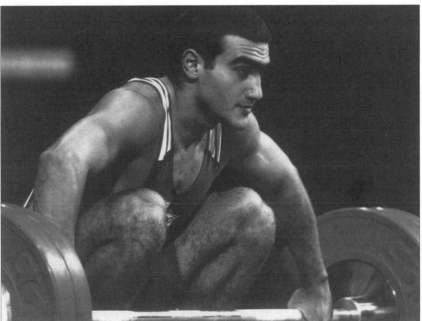

© Claus Andersen

Figure 4.4 Performance in some sports may benefit from a high degree of mental stimulation.

brain that influence emotions, such as arousal and relaxation, two important mental processes affecting sports performance.

Stimulation

Stimulation represents a state of arousal or motivation that may help enhance sports performance by optimizing neuromuscular functions. Stimulation techniques may benefit athletes in sports such as boxing or weightlifting (see figure 4.4).

Relaxation

Relaxation, a state of tranquility or calmness, may benefit athletes involved in sports such as archery in which excess arousal, anxiety, or stress may disrupt performance.

> **E**ven the most renowned athlete has doubts.
> — *Terry Orlick, sport psychologist*

MENTAL STRENGTH TRAINING

As noted, the human energy systems and support systems that generate physical power during exercise ultimately are controlled by the brain and spinal cord, collectively known as the central nervous system. Most of the neural control, or motor control, that enables your human energy systems to produce movement functions at a subconscious level. When you begin to jog, for example, hundreds of different muscles contract in rhythm, but you do not have to think about contracting each one at a specific time. Your nervous system calls each muscle into play at the appropriate time and controls the rate of energy production by the appropriate energy systems. The support systems for energy production are precisely regulated by the *autonomic nervous system,* a branch of the central nervous system. The rate and force of your heart contractions, as well as other body functions, adjust automatically to meet the demands of the exercise task. Thus, during such exercise as long-distance running you frequently can put your body on automatic pilot and think about other things.

On the other hand, there are many times in sport when you have to be conscious of what you are doing, such as when you are at bat awaiting a pitch. In such a situation, the motor control portion of your

Input	Interpretation	Output

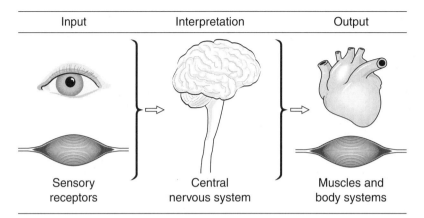

Sensory receptors	Central nervous system	Muscles and body systems

Figure 4.5 The nervous system receives information from various receptors, interprets this information in the central nervous system, and generates movement by muscular contraction.

brain must be functioning at an optimal level. It has to receive information, interpret it rapidly, and make a quick decision (see figure 4.5). There are three aspects to this process: (a) how effectively your senses receive the appropriate information or input, (b) how rapidly the analytical parts of your brain interpret this information, and (c) how accurately the motor control portion of your brain activates the proper muscles with the appropriate amount of force for optimal output. Any defect in the input or interpretation phase of this motor control process would lead to less than the optimal output.

Your brain controls virtually every physiological activity in your body. Although you rarely exercise its full potential, you can train it to an extraordinary degree. You can learn to control parts of your brain (including the autonomic nervous system) to the extent that you can lower your heart rate, decrease your blood pressure, increase blood flow to an area of your body, or change your skin temperature just by thinking about such developments. You also can train the motor control center in your brain to exert precise regulation of your muscular system. You can learn to make an individual muscle contract, enabling you, for instance, to wiggle your ears or move your middle toe only. Furthermore, many of the maneuvers in sports, such as those in rhythmic gymnastics, attest to the ability of the brain to control extremely complex muscular movement patterns.

The functioning of the motor control area, however, may be influenced by a part of the brain that you have not trained, or by neural feedback from other parts of the body. Your thoughts, your emotions, and your perceptions of bodily sensations experienced during sport competition can enhance or impair your performance. It is in this sense that we discuss the importance of the psychological state in sport; although the mind controls the body, the motor functions of the brain are susceptible to control by the emotional part of the brain.

Mental strength training, like physical power training, takes time to develop before an athlete receives any benefits. Since many of these mental training techniques have not been applied extensively to sport, some sport psychologists refer to them as *psychological sports ergogenics* when they are used in attempts to improve performance.

Everything may be in order physiologically for the athlete, but if the mind is not straight, the athlete will not perform optimally.

— *Terry Orlick, sport psychologist*

Psychological Sports Ergogenics as Training

As noted, you face a number of barriers in your attempts to achieve optimal performance in sport. Suppose your biceps muscle has the physiological potential to lift 400 pounds. That is, if your ATP-CP energy system could be maximally activated, the force developed would be transmitted to your forearm bone to move the weight. Such a force could prove to be excessive and could pull away a piece of the bone, a condition known as an *avulsion fracture*. Although avulsion fractures arise in sports such as weightlifting and arm wrestling, they are rare because of psychological limitations. Psychological barriers

---

Jerry Lynch, PhD, describes the case of Roger Bannister, the first human to break the 4-minute mile barrier. Lynch noted that by 1954 more than 50 medical journals had carried articles indicating it was humanly impossible to break 4 minutes in the mile. Bannister, however, believed he could, and he did break the 4-minute mile. Within about a year, four other runners broke the 4-minute barrier, suggesting the 4-minute mile was a mental barrier, not a physical one.

are built-in protective mechanisms that normally prevent you from reaching your full physiological potential. In this case your psychological limits may permit you to lift only 100 pounds.

Just as you have inherited a set of physical and physiological characteristics that may predispose you to success in a given sport, so too have you inherited a variety of psychological characteristics of similar value. Physical training can improve both physiological and psychological characteristics important to sport. Proper training, for example, will allow the lactic acid energy system in your muscles to produce more energy, but your psychological tolerance to pain also will increase, allowing you to accumulate more lactic acid in the blood before fatigue sets in. Your psychological limits have been raised, or in other words, you have increased your mental strength.

Psychological Sports Ergogenics and Arousal

Psychological sports ergogenics are designed to modify psychologic energy. For our purposes we will consider psychological energy to be the athlete's level of arousal, which may range from deep sleep to an extreme state of excitation. The *drive* and *inverted*-U theories are important relative to the application of arousal to sport performance.

The drive theory proposes that performance and arousal are directly related; as your level of arousal increases, so does your performance. This theory may be supported in athletic events that contain relatively basic, simple movement patterns, such as weightlifting. As illustrated in figure 4.6, the higher the degree of psychological energy, or arousal, the greater the strength potential.

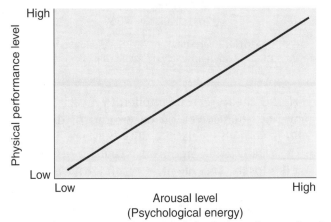

Figure 4.6 According to the drive theory of psychological arousal and physical performance, increased arousal will result in increased performance.

For sports that involve complex movement patterns and thought processes, the inverted-U theory presented in figure 4.7 may be more relevant. This theory proposes that there is an optimal level of arousal, which in figure 4.7 is theorized to be a moderate level. Arousal levels that are too low or too high might interfere with optimal performance. Members of a basketball team who read in the paper that their team is favored by 30 points might enter the game with a low level of arousal, believing all they have to do is show up. They might not get aroused until they are down by 10 points in the last few minutes of the game, but by then it's probably too late. On the other hand, if the same team were a 30-point underdog, the players might get so aroused that their high levels of anxiety would impair their ability to dribble and shoot the ball effectively.

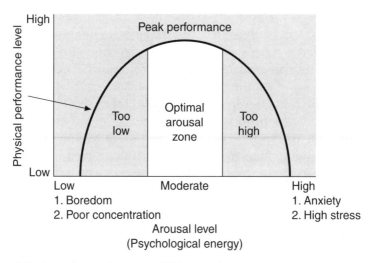

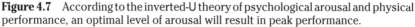

Figure 4.7 According to the inverted-U theory of psychological arousal and physical performance, an optimal level of arousal will result in peak performance.

The inverted-U theory can be applied to a variety of sports, and athletes may find themselves on either end of the U continuum. Athletes who have high levels of ability but face little challenge or demand are less likely to become aroused and more likely to be bored. They may suffer losses in concentration and drive and thus be more likely to suffer upsets in competition. On the other end of the continuum, athletes with ability levels much lower than the challenge they face are more likely to be aroused, often excessively so. The high anxiety and stress levels they experience can disrupt the ability to concentrate, increase muscle tension, and induce other physiological changes that might impair performance. Whenever the arousal level of the athlete is too low or too high, psychological ergogenic aids can be used to move athletes toward more optimal arousal levels, or zones, such as from high anxiety to relaxation during pistol shooting (figure 4.8).

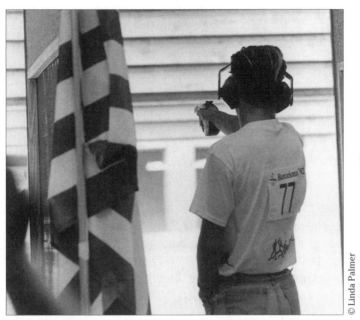

© Linda Palmer

Figure 4.8 Pistol shooting performance may be enhanced if the athlete can control excess anxiety and hand jitters through mental training techniques.

Optimal Arousal Zones

It is important to note that the optimal arousal zones may vary from sport to sport. Figure 4.9 represents theoretical curves for three sports: archery, tennis, and weightlifting. The optimal arousal zone for an archer might be low because any increase in muscle tension could result in impaired accuracy. Too little or too much arousal could adversely affect a tennis player's performance, so the optimal zone is in the middle. For weight training, the higher the arousal level the better, but there could be a point at which excessive anxiety could disrupt concentration.

The optimal arousal zone also varies from athlete to athlete. The curves in figure 4.9 could represent three batters. Each batter performs best at a different arousal level. The optimal arousal level for batter A is low, for batter B is medium, while batter C needs a high level of arousal.

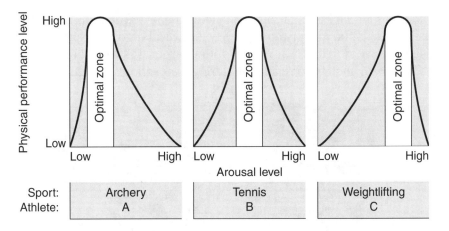

Figure 4.9 Differences might exist in optimal arousal zones for different sports or different athletes.

The key to psychological training techniques is to know your optimal arousal zone. For any athlete, this zone can change depending on the competition and the importance of the contest. It is important, therefore, that you know yourself and how you react to different levels of athletic competition. If you do, then the use of various psychological training techniques might help to improve your performance.

Mental Training Methods

As noted, one of the most effective ways to improve athletic performance is to improve physical power through proper physical training. A variety of training options are available, depending on the sport. For example, distance runners can use techniques such as interval training, repetition running, hill running, long-distance running, anaerobic threshold training, fartlek, and others.

A review of the sport psychology literature reveals a variety of mental training approaches or techniques, many of which are listed in table 4.2. Just as physical training is designed to maximize the positive aspects and minimize the negative aspects of physiological energy production, so does mental training attempt to maximize positive psychological energy and minimize negative psychological energy (figure 4.10).

Although physical training can help raise your psychological limits, it is theorized that psychological sports ergogenics might augment them even more. Psychotherapeutic techniques are designed to optimize mind functions (mental strength) during sport competition in the

---

TABLE 4.2
Mental Training Techniques

Attention control training	Mental dissociation
Attributional retraining	Mental rehearsal
Autogenic training	Negative thought stopping
Cognitive affective stress-management training	Positive thought control
	Progressive muscular relaxation
Cognitive restructuring	Rational emotive therapy
Concentration training	Relaxation training
Covert rehearsal techniques	Stress management
Flooding	Systematic desensitization
Flow	Sybervision
Goal setting	Transcendental meditation
Hypnosis	Visual motor behavior rehearsal
Imagery	Water flotation tanks
Implosive training	

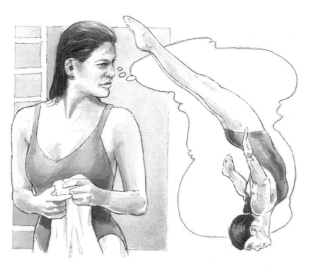

Figure 4.10 Mental imagery, or rehearsing sport skills in your mind, is one form of mental training.

---

way that physical training techniques are designed to optimize energy production (physical power).

The scope of this book does not permit a detailed discussion of the various mental strength training techniques that can be applied to sport. If you are interested in an expanded coverage, you might wish to read one or more of the excellent textbooks listed in the reference section. The books by Nideffer, Orlick, and Suinn are practical.

If you think you can't, you can't.

Many substances consumed by athletes to elicit a stimulant or calmative psychological effect will be covered in chapter 8.

Bill Roy, an Olympic hopeful in skeet shooting, was not able to spend time training as long or as often as others, so he attempted to make up for it with mental training. He would visualize a split-screen effect in which he pictured his body movements through his own eyes and from behind at the same time.

— *T. Kensler, writer for* Olympian

MENTAL STRENGTH AND FATIGUE

As noted, fatigue may occur because for various reasons the muscle is unable to generate physical power. Fatigue also may be caused by insufficient mental strength because various sites in the central or peripheral nervous system are not functioning optimally. Figure 4.11 shows some possible fatigue sites in the human body. The following discussion is keyed to the numbers in the figure.

1. One possible fatigue site is the motor nerve cells in the brain. The activity of these nerve cells is governed by various chemical neurotransmitters. Mental tiredness, lack of proper nutrition, and inhibition or inadequate stimulation from other parts of the brain may affect these neurotransmitters, limiting the ability to activate these motor neurons to their optimal potential. Conversely, overexcitability of motor neurons due to excess anxiety or stress might disrupt perceptual-motor skills, particularly fine motor control.

2. The motor nerve cell in the spinal cord leads directly to the muscle. This nerve cell may be inhibited by nerve centers in the brain, by various forms of feedback from the muscles, and by poor nutrition, thus leading to decreased work output.

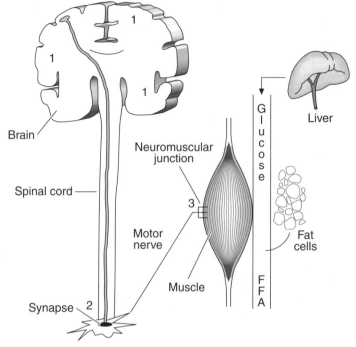

Figure 4.11 Possible fatigue sites in the nervous system (see text).

3. The junction of the nerve ending with the muscle cell can be a fatigue site if inadequate amounts of chemical neurotransmitters are secreted by the nerve ending or if the receptor on the muscle cell does not function properly. In such situations, an electrical impulse to initiate the contraction process would not be generated in the muscle cell.

SPORTS ERGOGENICS FOR MENTAL STRENGTH

Physical and mental preparation are important for success in athletic competition. In sport, the mind and body rely on each other for optimal functioning. What affects the body can affect the mind, and what affects the mind can affect the body.

If you can train your mind, your body will follow.

It is worth noting that some sports ergogenics designed to increase physical power SPFs might have some important implications for neural or psychological functioning during sport competition. Nutritional sports ergogenics, such as carbohydrate, can provide a source of muscle energy, but also might prevent the adverse psychological effects that low blood glucose levels have upon brain function. Pharmacological sports ergogenics, such as stimulants, can increase muscle metabolism, but also might directly stimulate brain function. Physiological sports ergogenics, such as sodium bicarbonate, may benefit metabolic processes in the muscle cells to help lessen psychological stress. Thus, some physical power sports ergogenics may improve sports performance by benefiting both physiological and psychological processes important to success.

Nutritional, pharmacological, and physiological sports ergogenics might be used because their purported effects on the nervous system are believed to help delay the onset of fatigue. Table 4.3 lists two general ways that sports ergogenics might be used in attempts to increase mental strength, and provides an example of specific nutritional, pharmacological, and physiological sports ergogenics that have been studied to determine their efficacy to induce such effects.

TABLE 4.3
Using Sports Ergogenics to Increase Mental Strength

1. To function as a stimulant, enhancing psychological functions that maximize energy production.

   Nutritional sports ergogenics: Amino acids

   Pharmacological sports ergogenics: Amphetamines

   Physiological sports ergogenics: Choline

2. To function as a calmative or depressant, reducing factors such as overexcitability or pain that may interfere with optimal psychological functioning.

   Nutritional sports ergogenics: B vitamins

   Pharmacological sports ergogenics: Narcotic analgesics

   Physiological sports ergogenics: Sodium bicarbonate

Chapter 6 lists nutritional, pharmacological, and physiological sports ergogenics that are theorized to increase mental strength SPFs by providing either a stimulant or calmative effect. Chapter 8 provides details relative to the effectiveness, safety, legal status, and ethics of these purported sports ergogenics.

5

GETTING A MECHANICAL ADVANTAGE

Sport involves the movement of matter. In some sports the main object moved is the body, which is a collection of different forms of matter such as bones, muscles, and fat. Running and high jumping are examples of sports in which we all want to move our bodies as fast or as high as we can. In these two sports, we also move other matter, such as the shoes and the uniform being worn.

Our primary goal in some other sports is to move matter other than our bodies at optimal speed, distance, or accuracy. External objects are used in many sports, each having its own characteristics as to the amount, type, and design of matter. Think of the dozens of different types of balls used for sports such as baseball, basketball, football, tennis, golf, soccer, field hockey, and jai alai; consider also the objects used in other sports, such as the javelin, shot, discus, hammer, arrow, and bullet. Although we give movement directly to many of these objects, we often need to move or control an object, such as a baseball bat, tennis racket, golf club, bow, or rifle, which imparts the force for movement. In still other sports the athlete controls an object that is the basis for participation, such as a bicycle, bobsled, horse, or sailboat.

MECHANICAL EDGE AND ENERGY

Remember the analogy of the racing car to physical power and mental strength presented previously? The engine generated physical power, or energy production, and a computerized fuel injection and steering system governed mental strength, or energy control. The mechanical edge, or energy efficiency, of a racing car is determined by its mechanics, including an optimal weight and a streamlined, aerodynamic design.

Mechanics is defined as the science of force and matter. It is the study of stationary and moving objects (matter) and the forces that cause them to move or to remain stationary. When applied to the study of humans and other living beings, this science is known as *biomechanics.* A subspecialty area of biomechanics is *sport biomechanics,* which involves the application of mechanical and biomechanical principles to the study of movement in sport.

Human Forces

Forces produce or stop motion. In chapter 3 we learned that human energy systems are designed to convert chemical energy to mechanical energy, resulting in force production through the mechanical energy created during muscular contraction. For many sports, we are interested in finding ways to maximize energy production, or physical power, to overcome physiological barriers and improve performance. We also are interested in ways to optimize energy control, or mental strength, to remove psychological barriers to optimal performance. We also want to optimize energy efficiency to provide a mechanical edge and to remove mechanical or biomechanical barriers. We do this by working with the forces of nature.

Natural Forces

From the viewpoint of obtaining a mechanical edge in sport, physical resistance to athletic performance provided by nature is of interest to us. In many sports we use our internal forces generated through muscle contraction to overcome some of the external forces in nature that resist movement. Although a variety of external forces exist in nature, those having the most significant effect on athletic performance are gravitational force, frictional force, forces found in moving fluids (both air and water are considered fluids by the physicist), buoyancy, and elasticity.

These forces may help to improve performance in some sports. An obvious example would be riding a bicycle downhill, a case in which the pulling force of gravity aids acceleration. Fluid forces such as a wind at the back of a cyclist or runner, or a following current for a triathlete in the swim portion of competition, provide additional forward force to increase speed. In some sports these forces are the basis for moving the athlete. Sky divers and downhill skiers rely on gravity to provide motion, while sailors rely on the wind and surfers depend on waves in water.

External forces usually provide resistance to movement in sport. Athletes who attempt to jump to great heights, such as high jumpers and pole vaulters, basically fight the force of gravity. Cyclists at high speeds face increased air resistance (see figure 5.1), while sprint swimmers experience high levels of water resistance. Increased frictional forces, such as the increased resistance of wet snow faced by a cross-country skier, might impede performance.

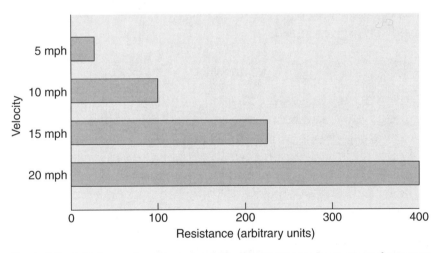

Figure 5.1 In high-speed events such as bicycling, resistance increases as the square of the velocity.

Techniques to obtain a mechanical edge are used to maximize any advantage that can be obtained from external forces or to minimize any adverse resistance effects. For sports that depend on external forces for motion, such as sailing, some research efforts have focused upon means to harness those forces more effectively, such as the design of better sails. Most of the research, however, has focused on reducing the resistive effects of gravitational pull, decreasing air and water resistance, and favorably modifying frictional forces, buoyancy, and elasticity.

MECHANICAL EDGE AND SPORT PERFORMANCE

Unlike nutrition, physiology, pharmacology, and psychology, mechanics is an exact science based upon proven laws of physics. The theoretical values of many sports ergogenics for physical power and mental strength are unsupported and need to be studied in rigorous research with athletes. This might be because individuals respond differently to these ergogenic aids. If we give 300 milligrams of caffeine to 10 different people, the magnitude of the physiological responses might be different in every subject. If we change the form of a bicycle helmet and measure the change in air resistance in a wind tunnel, however, we can predict rather precisely how much energy will be saved at any given speed.

T he 1989 Tour de France was a classic. The final stage involved a 15.5-mile (25-kilometer) time trial into Paris. Greg LeMond was in second place, 50 seconds behind Laurent Fignon, a time differential many believed was impossible to overcome. Both riders wore similar skintight suits and rode comparable bikes. LeMond, however, used an aerodynamic set of handlebars and an aerodynamic helmet; Fignon did not. Scientists have since concluded that those two modifications saved LeMond 1 minute and 16 seconds; he defeated Fignon by 8 seconds in the closest Tour de France finish ever.

Due to the exacting nature of the laws of physics, all forces known to affect performance can be manipulated in a variety of ways to predict the optimal body position, clothing, or sports equipment design for any given sport. Thus, much of the research associated with the development of a mechanical edge is simply the application of laws of physics to sport. Newton's Second Law of Motion, for example, deals with the interrelationships of force, mass, and acceleration. Acceleration of an object is directly proportional to the force applied to it and inversely proportional to its mass. All else being equal, a given force will produce greater acceleration of a lighter object than of a heavier one.

There are three general ways to obtain a mechanical edge in sport: (a) develop biomechanical skills specific to the sport, (b) use high-tech sportswear and sports equipment, and (c) modify body mass and body composition in accord with the demands of the sport. There are hundreds of specific applications of mechanical sports ergogenics, but space does not permit an extensive coverage, so only a brief description is offered for each area.

Mechanical Edge: Biomechanical Sport Skills

Improvement of biomechanical sport skills is one significant way of gaining a mechanical edge. You may have highly developed physical power, but if that energy or force is not applied to the desired movement in an effective and efficient manner, performance will not be optimal. You might have a powerful lactic acid energy system that gives you the potential to be an excellent 100-meter swimmer; if you do not have the necessary swimming skills, however, much of this energy potential will be wasted as you thrash your way down the pool.

Sport Skill Research

Researchers in sport biomechanics are constantly seeking ways to improve athletic performance by modifying how athletes apply their muscular forces to generate movement. These researchers have at their disposal an array of advanced technological equipment to record and analyze human movement. This equipment includes high-speed video cameras interfaced with computers to provide almost instantaneous analyses (figure 5.2). One of the major aims of biomechanical research is to develop specific sport skills so that the athlete's muscular energy forces are applied to movement in the most effective manner possible. Mechanical analyses of the arm pull in swimming and rowing, the leg and poling action in cross-country skiing, the sprint start in track, and arm and leg movements in the high-jump takeoff are examples of sports biomechanics research, the results of which may provide more effective techniques of applying force. Computerized analyses help adapt the skill to an individual athlete.

Decreasing resistance to movement is another major thrust of sports biomechanics research. Depending on the sport, research involving wind-tunnel tests suggests that a change in the position or surface area of a body might help to decrease resistance to movement.

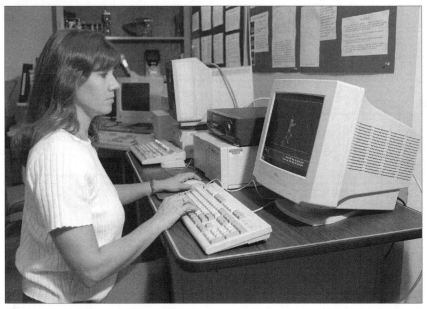

Figure 5.2 High-speed video cameras and computers provide instantaneous feedback on biomechanical analysis of various sport skills.

In high-speed sports such as bicycling, speed skating, downhill skiing, bobsledding, and luge, assuming a streamlined body position will help to decrease air resistance (figure 5.3). Such techniques become extremely important at high speeds, for nearly 90 percent of the resis-

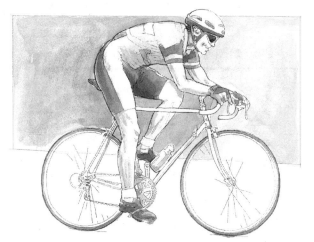

Figure 5.3 Modification of the body into a streamlined position helps reduce form drag.

tance to motion may be due to air resistance. Similar research using techniques that measure resistance in swimmers reveals that the position of the body in the water can be modified to reduce form drag and water resistance.

Sport Skill Improvement

Most methods to improve athletic performance through modification of body biomechanics are based on proper coaching and training. The development of the most efficient mechanical skills specific to a given sport, including how to maximize the application of force and minimize any resistant forces, occurs through sound analysis and the teaching of a knowledgeable coach. Many coaches, as well as tennis and golf professionals, also use high-speed video to improve the skills of their athletes. If such analyses are available, they might help you enhance your skill performance. Analysis and feedback from a knowledgeable coach or sports professional can be invaluable.

The scope of this book does not permit a detailed presentation of the biomechanics underlying the skills found in sports. Some excellent books cover sport biomechanics in general, while others focus upon the biomechanics of a specific sport. *The Biomechanics of Sports Techniques* by James Hay is an example of the former, while *Serious Cycling* by Edmund Burke is an example of the latter. A number of self-help resources also are available. Books specific to a given sport can provide current information on proper skill development. Films and videotapes of selected sport skills are commercially available.

Mechanical Edge: Sportswear and Sports Equipment

The sportswear and sports equipment industry is a multibillion-dollar business. Performance in almost every sport has been enhanced by technological advances in the design and manufacture of both sportswear and sports equipment.

Sportswear

All sports require some type of uniform, ranging from the brief suit of the male swimmer to the full wardrobe of the downhill skier. Wearing apparel designed specifically for athletes serves a variety of purposes, one of the most important being protection from the elements or from injury. Special fabrics enable runners to keep warm and dry while training in wet, cold conditions; modern running shoes balance cushioning and motion control to help prevent overuse injuries; and helmets can prevent serious head injury when accidents occur in high-speed and collision sports.

The type of sportswear that an athlete selects or is required to wear can affect performance. Virtually everything that athletes wear in competition has been modified in some way in attempts to improve performance. Helmets, glasses, uniforms, gloves, socks, and shoes have been engineered to save minutes, seconds, and even thousandths of a second in competition. Sportswear that provides a competitive edge over an opponent may be considered a mechanical ergogenic.

The design of sportswear for ergogenic purposes is based on the same principles of physics underlying modification of body biomechanics to improve performance. Depending upon the sport, sportswear may be engineered to decrease air resistance, water resistance, and gravitational forces; to increase or decrease friction and elasticity; or to increase buoyancy. Such effects could enhance athletic performance, as shown in the following examples.

Fluid Resistance. Research conducted in wind-tunnel tests conclusively shows that specially designed sportswear can reduce form drag or surface drag with a corresponding decrease in air resistance or water resistance. In high-speed sports such as downhill skiing, speed

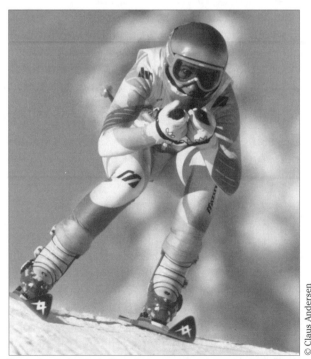

© Claus Andersen

Figure 5.4 Skintight uniforms help reduce air resistance at very high speeds in some sports.

skating, and bicycling, everything the athlete wears has been streamlined to make it more aerodynamic (figure 5.4). Streamlining the boots
used in downhill skiing may provide an advantage of less than a
second, but that could be the critical difference. The use of full-length,
skintight uniforms might help decrease air resistance at high speeds
by 6 to 10 percent, perhaps permitting a 4,000-meter pursuit bicyclist
to go 3 seconds faster. Formfitting swimsuits, especially for females,
have similar effects upon water resistance. Some research has suggested that the use of full torso swimsuits by male sprint swimmers
might decrease water resistance.

Buoyancy. Improved buoyancy would be advantageous to swimmers
because a higher body position in the water, with more of the body
moving through air, could reduce water resistance. In addition, less
energy would be expended to keep the body from sinking. There does not
appear to be any effective means of increasing buoyancy in most
swimming competition since flotation devices are illegal. Swimming is
one of the three events in the traditional triathlon, and these events often
are conducted at a time of the year when cold water temperature might
subject the athlete to a rapid loss of body heat. Use of wet suits could help
triathletes prevent hypothermia (excessively low body temperature),
but wet suits also give the swimmer additional buoyancy. If wet suits are
permitted, it might be a good idea to wear one; research suggests that
they might confer ergogenic benefits for most trained swimmers and
recreational triathletes. Australian investigators compared the times it
took trained swimmers to cover 1,500 meters, almost a mile, while
wearing three different suits: a wet suit, a Lycra triathlon suit, and an
ordinary swimsuit. The athletes' swim times while wearing the wet suits
were significantly faster than while wearing the other two suits, presumably due to the wet suits' buoyancy effect. Other research suggests that
elite swimmers who have perfected swimming mechanics would gain
very little benefit from wearing wet suits.

Gravity. Heavier sportswear could impair performance because it
would take more energy to overcome the additional gravitational
force. Thus, designers of athletic apparel use modern fabrics and
materials to provide the lightest sportswear possible for such sports.

Although most sportswear has benefited from such research and
design, sport shoes have received considerable attention. Any savings
in weight should be an advantage for an athlete who must move rapidly
for a long period of time. Several research studies support this point.
In one study, runners wearing shoes of different weights ran on a
treadmill at a set speed while their oxygen consumption was measured.

As expected, the runners' oxygen uptakes were higher while they were wearing heavier shoes, an indication that more energy was required than when the runners wore lighter shoes. Projected energy saving is about 0.28 percent for each ounce, so when a 5-ounce racing flat is substituted for a 10-ounce training shoe, the savings could cut several minutes from a racer's time in a long-distance races such as a marathon.

Other running shoes are designed to exploit energy storage and return associated with gravitational forces during running. With foot impact, gravitational forces are stored in special elastic materials used to construct the midsole and outsole of the shoe. This stored energy is returned to the foot on takeoff, reducing the oxygen demand of running and perhaps leading to improved performance.

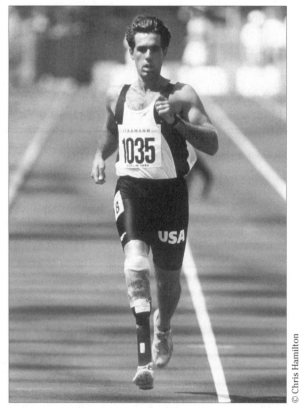

© Chris Hamilton

Figure 5.5 The lightweight high-tech materials now used in leg prostheses have significantly enhanced performance.

In Paralympic competition, high-tech materials such as carbon fiber and titanium have reduced the weight of leg prostheses for amputees by 10 to 15 pounds, enhancing performance accordingly.

Friction. In some sports the aim is to decrease friction, while in others it is to increase it. The smooth leather on the bottom of sliding-foot bowling shoes helps minimize friction forces and lets the bowler slide smoothly during delivery of the ball. In track events, the spikes on the shoes help to increase friction to prevent slipping, thus applying surface forces to help propel the athlete forward.

Appropriate sportswear can help athletes improve performance. Serious competitive athletes should stay abreast of technological developments and research findings regarding the application of sportswear modification to their sport. Many of these applications are reported in popular journals, such as *Bicycling* and *Runner's World*, that are available for almost every sport. Sportswear may be individually tailored for elite athletes at the international level of competition.

Sports Equipment

For the purpose of this discussion, sports equipment is differentiated from sportswear. We shall consider sports equipment to be any ball, instrument, or vehicle essential to the conduct of the sport. A basic premise of sport is that an equipment advantage should not be instrumental in deciding the outcome of the contest. This is no problem in sports such as swimming, for basically no equipment is used. In other sports, such as cycling, equipment is crucial to the outcome and a superior design might provide an advantage.

In attempts to make competition equal among participating athletes, all sports have rules governing various aspects of sports equipment, such as weight, dimensions, and design. Although design engineers can do little to improve some equipment—such as the 16-pound shot, which is not very aerodynamic—in others they can make remarkable changes that will improve performance. For example, older rules for the javelin stipulated its weight and length but said little of its design. Consequently, engineers designed an aerodynamic javelin that could be thrown well beyond 300 feet, which in some competition sites put it in the stands with the spectators, many of whom did not consider this a good example of a spectator sport. The rules subsequently were changed to include limitations on the javelin's design.

Although sports equipment is designed for a variety of purposes, such as comfort and safety, from an ergogenic standpoint the major purpose is to improve athletic performance by providing a mechanical edge. Some sports allow for some leeway in equipment design; the advent of *computer-assisted design (CAD)* has transformed the process of designing sports equipment. Because the mathematical laws of physics are immutable, variables such as weight, size, wind velocity, and others can be entered into a computer program and manipulated until optimal results are obtained. Thus, sport technologists may be able to provide athletes with a competitive advantage by modifying the equipment to take advantage of fluid, buoyancy, gravity, and friction forces (figure 5.6).

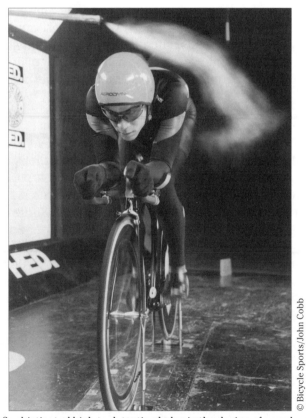

© Bicycle Sports/John Cobb

Figure 5.6 Sophisticated high-tech testing helps in the design of aerodynamic sport equipment.

There are several basic categories of equipment used in sports. Objects such as balls, javelins, and arrows are propelled for distance or accuracy. Implements such as tennis rackets, lacrosse sticks, and bows are used to receive objects and to impart or control the application of force to objects. Other equipment transports the athlete; in some cases the athlete provides most of the force for movement, such as to bicycles and cross-country skis. In other cases the athlete is primarily responsible for controlling movement of a vehicle, such as a bobsled or sailboat, the movement of which is produced by gravity or wind. A major goal of engineers is to improve the effectiveness of the various types of sports equipment to fulfill their basic functions optimally. Some examples follow.

Sports Objects. If the purpose of a sport is to propel an object for distance or accuracy, then the object itself can be modified to achieve these objectives. Changing the shape and composition of the object may affect its speed, distance, and accuracy. The distance the javelin could be thrown was improved markedly by adding an aerodynamically designed flattened tail section that provided a greater lifting effect. Golf balls fly a greater distance given modifications to the number and configuration of dimples in the ball. In archery, arrows can be designed to fly truer to the target. Numerous examples could be cited, but in most sports the characteristics of the object are restricted and not subject to modification.

Sports Implements. Sports implements used to impart movement to the human body or other objects have received much research attention. The results of such research have led to significant improvements in athletic performance. One example is the fiberglass pole used in pole vaulting. Vaulters using aluminum poles tried for years to break the elusive 15-foot barrier and finally succeeded. Immediately after the fiberglass pole became available, however, vaulters easily scaled this former barrier, and the world record is now over 20 feet (see figure 5.7).

The composition of an implement might influence its striking characteristics. Research shows that an aluminum bat may impart more speed to a baseball than a wooden bat. This finding was attributed to the uniform distribution of material in the hollow aluminum bat compared to a less uniform density in the wooden bat. In essence, the more uniform composition provided a more effective center of percussion, resulting in less vibration or wasted energy upon impact and hence more speed; the *center of percussion* is the so-called *sweet spot.*

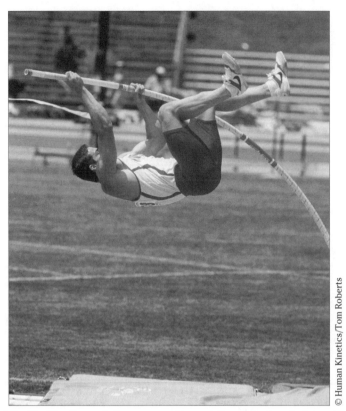

© Human Kinetics/Tom Roberts

Figure 5.7 Modification of the composition of the pole has led to significant improvements in pole vaulting performance.

One advantage of larger heads in tennis racquets is the increased sweet spot. Golf clubs and other striking implements also may be designed along these lines.

Sports Vehicles. Engineers have markedly improved the mechanics of sports equipment used to move the athlete, such as the bobsled, luge, skis, sailboat, and bicycle. Most of the research has focused on means of reducing resistances, both fluid and frictional. Modifications in the design of the bicycle illustrate how decreasing resistance can improve performance. An elite competitor's bicycle is lightweight due to special metal alloys, is aerodynamically designed from the seat down to the water bottle, is equipped with wheels and tires specifically designed to minimize air and rolling resistance, and may be tailored to the specific body configurations of the cyclist. Such bicycles can cost $30,000 or more (see figure 5.8).

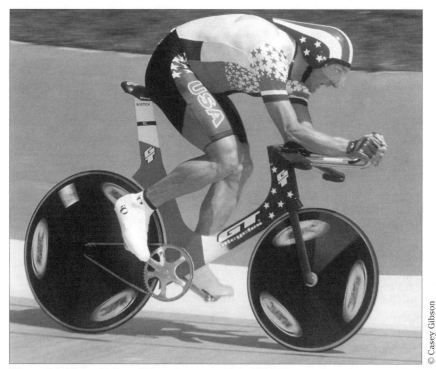

© Casey Gibson

Figure 5.8 Some high-tech bicycles cost nearly $30,000.

Our general recommendation regarding sports equipment is comparable to the one we offered on the use of sportswear. You need to be aware of changes in equipment design brought about by research and technology. Again, popular magazines for specific sports often focus on advancements that appear to be supported by sound logic and research.

Elite athletes need to be assured that they have the best equipment available. If not, they will be at a definite mechanical disadvantage, and possibly a psychological disadvantage if they know their opponents have better equipment. Although equipment disparity usually is not that great at this level of competition, there have been situations in which it could mean the difference between winning and losing.

Technology can take you only so far, but all other things being equal, it can take you farther or faster than your opponent.

For the everyday athlete, training is still the key to improved performance. You may be as well trained a triathlete as the person next to you, but if you show up with your old Columbia one-speed with balloon tires and your opponent has an $8,000 customized Trek, it's a pretty safe bet who will win the bike phase of the competition.

If you are a serious competitor and want to be all that you can possibly be, then you can buy technology to enhance your performance. As with most things in life, however, the best usually costs more, so the amount of mechanical edge you can buy may depend on the size of your wallet.

Mechanical Edge: Body Height, Type, Mass, and Composition

Just as the genes you inherited from your parents may provide you with physiological and psychological characteristics essential for athletic success, they also have provided you with a unique set of morphological characteristics that might predispose you to success in some sports, but limit your ability in others. Body height, body type, body mass, and body composition are morphological characteristics that might provide a mechanical edge in some sports.

Body height may be beneficial in some sports, such as in the high jump. The taller athlete has a higher center of gravity, and thus does not have to raise it as far to clear the bar compared to a shorter competitor. In contrast, a shorter athlete will have an advantage in the high bar, a gymnastic event, because of a greater strength relative to body size. Bone length and width may be important as well. Individuals with long arms may be more successful in throwing a discus, while those with shorter arms may have an advantage in weightlifting. Narrow hips might give female sprint runners an advantage.

> **D**escription of Tom Dolan, an Olympic swimmer: "He is as long and lean as an eel. His arms stretch to hands that look like canoe paddles, and if his feet were any bigger, they could be classified as paddles."
>
> — *Gerry Callahan,* Sports Illustrated *writer*

Body type (body shape or *somatotype*) may be an important aspect of various sports competitions. Although a wide range of body types might be successful in any given sport, research conducted with athletes has revealed that certain body types tend to gravitate toward specific sports or positions in sports. For example, most elite distance runners have relatively lean body frames, most weight lifters are highly muscular, and most sumo wrestlers are somewhat obese. In the sport of bodybuilding, body type and muscularity is the focus of competition. In some sports, such as gymnastics, figure skating, and diving, the body type and shape might not be the major focus of the competition, but it might influence the evaluation of performance from an aesthetic standpoint.

Body mass represents the body weight, and body composition the relative amount of body fat and lean body mass (which is mainly muscle tissue). Body mass in itself might confer an advantage in sports such as sumo wrestling, in which stability is important. Increased body mass, particularly lean body muscle mass, might enhance power production, an important consideration for athletes in strength-power sports such as weightlifting. Conversely, excess body mass, particularly body fat, might be a disadvantage to athletes such as gymnasts and distance runners, who need to lift or move their bodies (figure 5.9).

You can do little to change your body height or your bone structure, but through training you can change several biomechanical aspects of your body, possibly resulting in improved performance.

Weight Control and Mechanical Edge

For many sports, one biomechanical means that might give you a mechanical edge is adjustment of your body mass. Decreasing body weight can reduce the effect of gravitational pull and might be helpful in sports such as gymnastics, in which the body weight needs to be supported. Increasing body weight increases gravitation pull and friction on the body, and may be an important way for sumo wrestlers and interior linemen in American football to resist movement.

Theoretical considerations and research suggest that the composition of your body may significantly affect your performance in sports. Your body weight is related to a variety of tissues, but for this discussion we will consider only two major components: body fat and lean body mass. Most of your lean body mass consists of muscle tissue, which is approximately 70 percent water. Thus, water can be considered a third component of your body weight. Although research has not revealed a specific percentage of body fat or lean body mass to be ideal for any given sport, enough scientific data exists to make some generalizations.

Weight Loss. In general, research supports the finding that excess body fat might impair performance in sports in which the body needs

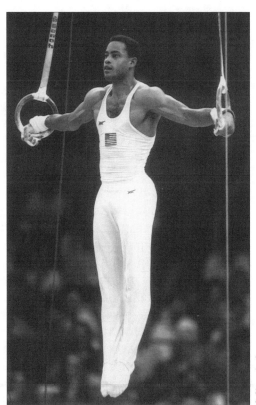

Figure 5.9 Low body mass and fat may provide a biomechanical edge in some sports, such as gymnastics, while increased body and muscle mass may be biomechanically advantageous for other sports, such as sumo wrestling.

© Claus Andersen

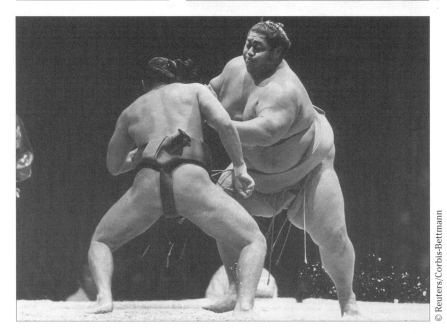

© Reuters/Corbis-Bettmann

to be moved rapidly or efficiently, such as high jumping or long-distance running. Epidemiological research reveals low body fat percentages in such athletes as distance runners, high jumpers, gymnasts, ballet dancers, sprinters, and others for whom excess body fat could be a disadvantage. Experimental studies in which weights mimicking body fat were strapped to the bodies of runners demonstrated a decrease in efficiency when running. Such research findings in sport reflect the basic laws of physics; more energy is required to move a greater mass against the force of gravity. Although a certain amount of body fat is necessary for optimal health and physiological functioning, too much fat is excess baggage. Research involving physiological measurements has suggested that a 160-pound (72.5-kilogram) male runner could expect to improve performance by about 6 minutes in a 26.2-mile (42.2-kilometer) marathon if he were to lose 5 percent of his body weight, the equivalent of 8 pounds (3.6 kilograms)of fat.

Losing excess body fat, which may be accomplished safely by proper dietary adjustments, will improve energy efficiency because less weight needs to be moved.

Research has shown that slow weight losses resulting from exercise and moderate restriction of caloric intake will help an athlete maintain performance capacity. Lean muscle mass may be maintained by a properly designed weight-training program. Thus, a proper weight-reduction program can be an effective way to improve performance in certain sports.

Improper weight-loss programs, however, could impair the health of athletes. Some athletes, particularly females in weight-control sports, develop disordered eating patterns that can have serious consequences. In the female athlete triad, disordered eating might lead to hormonal imbalances, amenorrhea, and disturbances in bone metabolism. Such athletes are at increased risk for stress fractures and premature osteoporosis (a significant decrease in bone density). Sports medicine professionals have reported that some female athletes in their 20s have bone mineral densities of women in their 60s.

Some weight-loss strategies, such as excessive dehydration, rapid starvation, and the use of laxatives and diuretics, could impair various types of sports performance. When carried to extremes, unsupervised excessive weight loss could be fatal.

According to sports officials, South Korean Chung Se-hoon, a gold medal hopeful at the 1996 Olympic Games, died of a heart attack apparently brought on by a crash diet. He was on a diet to lose 18 pounds to meet a weight check for judo team members.

Weight Gain. Increased body weight may be an advantage in some sports. In contact sports such as American-style or Australian-style football, ice hockey, and sumo wrestling, a greater body mass might help the athlete maintain stability and resist forces generated by opponents. Although a little additional body fat might be useful in such sports, the increased body weight should be primarily in the form of muscle tissue. Research with professional football players, even many interior linemen, reveals relatively low levels of body fat and high muscularity. Moreover, literally hundreds of weight-training studies have shown that increases in muscle mass usually are accompanied by increases in strength, power, and performance.

Through weight training . . . everything I put on is muscle in the upper body. The stronger I am in my upper body, the better I am able to hold my form. That's one reason my 400 time has improved.

— *Michael Johnson, first male Olympian to win both the 200- and 400-meter races*

Proper Weight Loss and Gain. In any weight-control program, whether the goal is to lose or gain weight, it is important to follow sound principles of nutrition. In general you should not lose more than 2 pounds per week unless under medical supervision. A deficit of 1,000 calories per day will result in the loss of about 2 pounds per week; such a deficit can be achieved by expending 500 calories per day through exercise, and decreasing food intake by 500 calories. The amount of exercise necessary to burn 500 calories is the approximate equivalent of running 5 miles. Reducing the amount of fat and sugar in your diet is usually all that is necessary to save 500 dietary calories per day.

Gaining weight in the form of muscle mass requires a proper

resistance-training program with weights, such as free weights or machines, and an additional 400–500 calories daily. A gain of about 1 pound per week appears to be a realistic goal on such a program. Ask your physician or a local sport nutritionist to recommend sensible programs for weight control.

MECHANICAL EDGE AND FATIGUE

As noted in chapters 3 and 4, fatigue may be caused by the inability to produce adequate physical power or mental strength to control that power. Fatigue also may be caused by an insufficient mechanical edge. Poor mechanics or biomechanics in sport, such as the following, results in inefficient movement that will predispose an athlete to premature fatigue.

1. Inferior biomechanical sport skills will impair the application of propulsive forces to movement and/or the ability to overcome resistive forces to movement.
2. The use of substandard sportswear and equipment in a specific sport will result in wasted application of physical power.
3. Excess accumulation of body mass, particularly body fat, might impose a mechanical disadvantage because it normally costs more energy to move the additional mass, which in itself does not augment energy production during exercise. Conversely, inadequate body mass, particularly muscle mass, can be a disadvantage in sports in which increased body stability is important.

SPORTS ERGOGENICS FOR MECHANICAL EDGE

Appropriate training to improve biomechanical sport skills and to favorably modify body composition is an important way to obtain a mechanical edge, as is the use of appropriate sportswear and sports equipment, but technically these are not sports ergogenics.

As noted in table 5.1, nutritional, pharmacological, and physiological sports ergogenics have been used to modify body mass and composition.

Chapter 6 lists nutritional, pharmacological, and physiological sports ergogenics that have been purported to increase mechanical

> **TABLE 5.1**
> Using Sports Ergogenics to Increase Mechanical Edge
>
> 1. Increase body mass or muscle mass.
>   Nutritional sports ergogenics: Amino acids
>   Pharmacological sports ergogenics: Anabolic steroids
>   Physiological sports ergogenics: Creatine
> 2. Decrease body mass or fat mass.
>   Nutritional sports ergogenics: Chromium
>   Pharmacological sports ergogenics: Diuretics
>   Physiological sports ergogenics: Human growth hormone

edge primarily by helping the athlete gain muscle mass or decrease body fat. Chapter 8 provides details relative to the effectiveness, safety, legal aspects, and ethics of these purported sports ergogenics.

EXAMINING PERFORMANCE FACTORS IN SPECIFIC SPORTS

Each sport has inherent, specific sports performance factors (SPFs) relative to physical power, mental strength, and mechanical edge. Some sports require high power, others low power. Some sports benefit from increased arousal, others from relaxation. Some sports benefit greatly from improved mechanics, others to a lesser extent.

Sports ergogenics are designed to improve specific SPFs. Some are effective, others are not.

This chapter will help you determine the SPFs that are inherent to your sport, and help you identify sports ergogenics that have been purported to enhance those SPFs.

SPORTS PERFORMANCE FACTORS (SPFs)

Most sports involve a complex array of SPFs that are associated with successful performance. Taking a holistic approach, each SPF (including multiple subdivisions) involved in a particular sport would be identified and analyzed regarding its relative importance and contribution to success. Successful performance is the sum of the contributions from all specific SPFs.

> The Australian rowing federation worked with coaches and sport scientists to develop a profile of women athletes who had the potential to become world-class rowers.
> — *Jay Kearney, senior sports physiologist, USOC*

Using a reductionist approach, we identify important SPFs but simplify the process by attempting to group specific SPFs into several general categories. Although we may lose some specificity with this approach, it appears to be appropriate for identifying those primary SPFs that might be influenced by sports ergogenics. Table 6.1 presents the general SPFs for physical power, mental strength, and mechanical edge that may be influenced by sports ergogenics; an expanded discussion of the SPFs in each of these three general categories is presented in chapters 3, 4, and 5, respectively. A brief review in the following sections uses running events as illustrative examples.

TABLE 6.1
Sports Performance Factors

Physical power (energy production)
Explosive power and strength
High power and speed
Power endurance
Aerobic power
Aerobic endurance

Mental strength (neuromuscular control)
Stimulation
Relaxation

Mechanical edge (efficiency)
Increased muscle/body mass
Decreased body fat/body mass

Physical Power

Explosive strength and power represent the ability to produce force very rapidly. Explosive strength, often referred to as explosive power, is the ability to use dynamic strength very rapidly (a second or so), such as for a sprint start in a 100-meter dash. Explosive strength also may involve static or isometric strength, such as in an initial stalemate phase of arm wrestling. ATP is the primary energy source used to generate explosive strength or power.

High power, or speed, represents the ability to produce force very rapidly, but for somewhat longer periods of time (5–30 seconds) compared to explosive power. Speed is anaerobic power. In track, 100- and 200-meter dash performance depends on speed. It might be necessary to maintain high levels of static strength for similar time frames. CP is a primary energy source used to generate speed and high levels of static strength.

Power endurance, or anaerobic endurance, is the ability to sustain high levels of muscle force development for about 45 seconds to 2 minutes, such as in running a 400- or 800-meter race. Prolonged intermittent high power production, as in soccer, may lead to progressive increases in lactic acid, which could reflect a form of power endurance. Muscle glycogen is the primary energy source used by the FT muscle fiber to generate power endurance.

Aerobic power is the ability to utilize oxygen at a high percentage of maximal. Such events may last 13–30 minutes or so. Running events such as 5–10 kilometers (3.1–6.2 miles) depend on aerobic power. Muscle glycogen is the primary energy source used by the ST muscle fiber, and some FT muscle fibers, to generate aerobic power.

Aerobic endurance is the ability to generate force from oxidative processes at a lower percent of VO_2max compared to aerobic power, but is sustainable for hours such as in marathons (42.2 kilometers, 26.2 miles) and ultramarathons (100 kilometers, 62.2 miles). Muscle glycogen, blood glucose, muscle triglycerides, and plasma free fatty acids serve as energy sources.

Mental Strength

Stimulation represents the ability to arouse the nervous system, enhancing psychological functions such as reaction time, visual acuity, and complex muscle coordination that may maximize energy production. Stimulation might decrease the time it takes to respond to the sound of the starting gun in a 100-meter dash.

Relaxation, or depression, represents the ability to calm the nervous system. A calmative effect may reduce factors such as overexcitability or pain that might interfere with optimal psychological function and energy production. Relaxation might help the jittery 100-meter sprinter avoid a false start at the beginning of the race.

Mechanical Edge

An increased body mass, primarily muscle mass but also body fat for some sports, represents an increased ability to resist external forces designed to move the body, as observed in the increased stability of a 200-kilogram (440-pound) sumo wrestler. Increased muscle mass, if it improves energy production, might help sprinters. But increased body mass, particularly fat, generally will impair aerobic power and endurance.

A decreased body mass, particularly body fat, represents an increased ability to reduce resistance to muscular forces designed to move the body, as observed in the increased efficiency of the lean distance runner.

SPORT AND SPORTS PERFORMANCE FACTORS

Success in any sport may depend on a variety of physiological, psychological, and biomechanical SPFs. Determination of the predominant SPF is less difficult for some sports than for others. For example, a competitive weight lifter needs explosive power, a high level of stimulation, and an increased muscle mass. A competitive decathlete or heptathlete, on the other hand, needs a greater diversity of SPFs, including explosive power, high power or speed, power endurance, and aerobic power; a stimulant effect might enhance performance in some events, while a calmative effect might benefit others. The same, respectively, could be said for an increased and a decreased body mass.

Table 6.2 indicates the general SPFs for athletes participating in a variety of sports and sport events. Other SPFs may be important, but the designated SPFs are those believed to be most relevant. To use table 6.2, find your sport and note the corresponding SPFs that are thought to be important.

The following points should be kept in mind relative to the three major SPF classifications: physical power, mental strength, and mechanical edge.

TABLE 6.2
Sports and Sports Performance Factors

SPORT	PHYSICAL POWER					MENTAL STRENGTH		MECHANICAL EDGE	
	Explosive power	High power	Power endurance	Aerobic power	Aerobic endurance	Stimulation	Relaxation	Lose fat	Gain muscle
Archery							X		
Athletics (see Field events, Track events)									
Auto racing						X			
Badminton	X	X		X		X			
Baseball	X	X				X		X	X
Basketball	X	X	X			X		X	X
Biathlon (riflery, cross-country skiing)				X			X	X	
Bicycling Sprint Pursuit		X	X			X		X	
Bicycling Road racing Time trial				X	X	X		X	
Billiards							X		
Bobsledding	X	X				X			

(continued)

TABLE 6.2 (continued)
Sports and Sports Performance Factors

SPORT	PHYSICAL POWER					MENTAL STRENGTH			MECHANICAL EDGE	
	Explosive power	High power	Power endurance	Aerobic power	Aerobic endurance	Stimulation	Relaxation		Lose fat	Gain muscle
Bodybuilding, competitive	X								X	X
Bowling							X			
Boxing						X			X	
Canoeing/ kayaking Flatwater Whitewater			X			X				
Cricket	X	X				X				
Dancing, competitive aerobic			X	X		X			X	
Decathlon (shot, discus, javelin, long jump, high jump, pole vault, 100-m dash, 110-m hurdles, 400-m, 1,500-m run)	X	X	X	X		X	X		X	X

(continued)

Sport							
Diving							
Platform			X				X
Springboard							
Equestrian			X				X
Fencing		X		X			X
Field events, jumping							
High jump				X			X
Long jump							
Triple jump							
Pole vault							
Field events, throwing							
Discus	X			X			X
Hammer							
Javelin							
Shot							
Field hockey		X		X	X	X	
Fishing, deep sea				X	X		
Football, American							
Lineman	X			X		X	
Linebacker							
Football, American							
Offensive back		X		X		X	
Defensive back							
Football, Australian rules		X		X		X	

TABLE 6.2 (continued)
Sports and Sports Performance Factors

SPORT	PHYSICAL POWER					MENTAL STRENGTH		MECHANICAL EDGE	
	Explosive power	High power	Power endurance	Aerobic power	Aerobic endurance	Stimulation	Relaxation	Lose fat	Gain muscle
Golf	X						X		
Gymnastics High bar Pommel horse Rings Uneven bars	X	X					X	X	
Gymnastics Balance beam Floor routine Vault	X						X	X	
Handball	X	X				X			
Heptathlon (shot, javelin, long jump, high jump, 200-m dash, 100-m hurdles, 800-m run)	X	X	X			X		X	X
Horse racing Thoroughbred						X			
Ice hockey	X	X				X			X

Activity								
Lacrosse	X		X			X	X	X
Luge		X	X					X
Martial arts Jujitsu Judo Karate	X		X					X
Motorboat racing								
Motorcycling Motocross			X					
Mountain climbing	X		X	X	X			X
Orienteering	X		X	X	X			X
Pentathlon (Fencing, riding, running, shooting, swimming)		X	X	X	X	X		X
Polo	X		X					
Racket sports Paddleball Racquetball Squash Table tennis	X	X	X				X	X
Rowing (2,000-m)	X		X		X			X
Rugby	X	X	X					X

(continued)

89

TABLE 6.2 (*continued*)
Sports and Sports Performance Factors

SPORT	PHYSICAL POWER					MENTAL STRENGTH		MECHANICAL EDGE	
	Explosive power	High power	Power endurance	Aerobic power	Aerobic endurance	Stimulation	Relaxation	Lose fat	Gain muscle
Running (See also Track) Marathon (42.2 km, 26.2 mi) Ultramarathons (50 km & beyond)					X			X	
Sailing, yachting		X				X			
Shooting Pistol Rifle							X		
Skating, ice 500–1,500 m Short track			X			X		X	
Skating, ice 5,000–10,000 m				X		X		X	
Skating, figure	X						X	X	
Ski jumping	X						X		

Activity								
Skiing, snow Downhill racing Slalom			X		X			
Skiing, snow Cross-country (Nordic)		X	X	X	X		X	
Soccer Forwards Defense	X				X		X	
Soccer Goalie	X				X			
Swimming, sprint 100–200 m			X		X			
Swimming, endurance 400–1,500 m Open water swims				X	X			
Swimming, synchronized				X		X		
Surfing	X				X			
Sumo wrestling	X				X			X
Track events 100–200 m		X			X		X	
Track events 400–800 m	X				X		X	
Track events 5,000–10,000 m				X	X		X	

(continued)

TABLE 6.2 (continued)
Sports and Sports Performance Factors

SPORT	PHYSICAL POWER					MENTAL STRENGTH		MECHANICAL EDGE	
	Explosive power	High power	Power endurance	Aerobic power	Aerobic endurance	Stimulation	Relaxation	Lose fat	Gain muscle
Triathlon (swim 1 km, bike 40 km, run 10 km)				X		X		X	
Ultraendurance events					X			X	
Volleyball	X					X		X	
Walking, competitive 20–50 km				X	X			X	
Water polo	X		X	X		X			
Water skiing						X			
Weightlifting, competitive	X					X		X	X
Wrestling Freestyle Greco-Roman	X	X				X		X	

Physical power. Many sport activities involve a blend of energy production from the three energy systems. Racing 200 meters, for example, involves all three energy systems, but the ATP-CP energy system predominates. In some sports, such as the decathlon, multiple energy systems are needed. More than one physical power SPF may be checked for some sports.

Mental strength. Stimulation is the predominant mental strength SPF for most sports, but relaxation may be helpful in those sports where anxiety might disrupt performance. The effect of stimulation or relaxation may depend on the individual athlete. Gymnasts probably would benefit most from a stimulation effect; for a highly anxious gymnast, however, excess stimulation might impair performance, while relaxation techniques could reduce anxiety and help the athlete reach an optimal level of arousal.

Mechanical edge. In most sports, athletes wish to increase muscle mass and decrease body fat. With the possible exception of a few sports, such as sumo wrestling and long-distance swimming, decreased body fat will increase performance, all other things being equal. Increased muscle mass increases the potential to increase physical power, but might also increase the mass, or resistance, to movement. Increased upper-body muscle mass might help the decathlete in some events, such as the shot put, but could be a handicap in others, such as the 1,500-meter run.

Athletes should be aware of the SPFs inherent to their sport, keeping in mind that the SPFs indicated in table 6.2 may need to be modified for them.

SPORTS PERFORMANCE FACTORS AND SPORTS ERGOGENICS

Table 6.3 lists all the sports ergogenics covered in chapter 8 and the five SPFs for physical power, the two SPFs for mental strength, and the two SPFs for mechanical edge. To use table 6.3, find the SPFs important to your sport in table 6.2, and then in table 6.3 locate sports ergogenics theorized to enhance those SPFs, as indicated by the X in that column.

Please note that the X indicates only that the sport ergogenic has been linked theoretically to the SPF and that some research has been conducted to evaluate the efficacy of the sport ergogenic to improve that SPF or some related sport performance. It is important to note that the X does *not* mean the sport ergogenic is effective.

TABLE 6.3
Sports Ergogenics and Sports Performance Factors

SPORTS ERGOGENIC	PHYSICAL POWER					MENTAL STRENGTH		MECHANICAL EDGE	
	Explosive power	High power	Power endurance	Aerobic power	Aerobic endurance	Stimulation/ arousal	Relaxation/ reduce pain	Lose fat/ body mass	Gain muscle/ body mass
Alcohol							X		
Amphetamines	X	X	X	X	X	X		X	
Anabolic phytosterols	X	X	X					X	X
Anabolic/ androgenic steroids	X	X	X					X	X
Antioxidants	X	X	X	X	X				
Arginine, lysine, ornithine	X	X	X					X	X
Aspartates		X	X	X	X				
Bee pollen				X					
Beta-blockers							X		
Beta-2 agonists	X	X	X	X		X			X
Blood doping				X	X				
Boron	X	X	X					X	X

Branched-chain amino acids (BCAA)					X		
Caffeine		X	X	X	X		
Calcium	X	X	X	X			
Carbohydrate supplements		X	X	X			
Carnitine		X	X	X			
Choline				X			
Chromium	X	X		X		X	X
Cocaine	X	X	X	X	X		
Coenzyme Q$_{10}$			X	X			
Creatine				X			X
Dehydroepiandrosterone (DHEA)	X	X				X	X
Diuretics	X	X				X	
Engineered dietary supplements		X				X	X
Ephedrine	X	X	X	X	X	X	
Erythropoietin	X	X	X	X			
Fat supplementation				X			
Fluid supplementation				X	X		

(continued)

TABLE 6.3 (continued)
Sports Ergogenics and Sports Performance Factors

SPORTS ERGOGENIC	PHYSICAL POWER					MENTAL STRENGTH		MECHANICAL EDGE	
	Explosive power	High power	Power endurance	Aerobic power	Aerobic endurance	Stimulation/ arousal	Relaxation/ reduce pain	Lose fat/ body mass	Gain muscle/ body mass
Folic acid				X	X				
Ginseng		X	X	X	X				
Glycerol				X	X				
HMB	X	X	X					X	X
Human growth hormone	X	X	X					X	X
Inosine	X	X		X	X				
Iron				X	X				
Magnesium	X			X	X				X
Marijuana						X	X		
Multivitamin/ mineral supplements	X	X	X	X	X		X		X
Narcotic analgesics							X		
Niacin			X	X	X				
Nicotine	X	X	X	X	X	X			

Supplement	Col 1	Col 2	Col 3	Col 4	Col 5	Col 6	Col 7	Col 8
Omega-3 fatty acids	X			X	X			
Oxygen supplementation				X	X	X		
Pantothenic acid				X	X			
Phosphates	X			X	X	X		X
Protein supplements						X		X
Riboflavin				X	X			
Selenium				X	X			
Sodium bicarbonate						X		
Testosterone and human chorionic gonadotropin	X	X				X		X
Thiamin			X	X	X	X		
Tryptophan			X		X	X		
Vanadium	X			X	X			X
Vitamin B$_6$	X		X	X	X	X		X
Vitamin B$_{12}$	X		X	X	X	X		X
Vitamin B$_{15}$				X	X			
Vitamin C				X	X	X		
Vitamin E				X	X	X		
Yohimbine	X	X			X			X
Zinc	X				X			X

If you are interested in what research indicates regarding the effectiveness of a specific sport ergogenic, that information can be found in chapter 8. Information is also presented relative to the safety, legal status, and ethical concerns of the sport ergogenic, along with general recommendations regarding its use by athletes to improve sport performance.

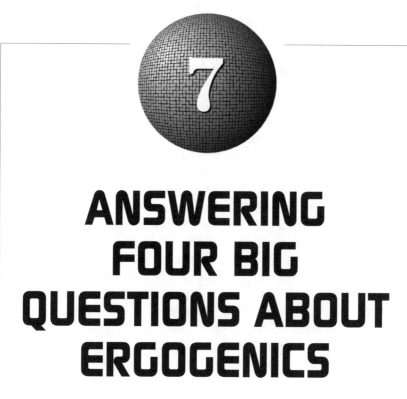

ANSWERING FOUR BIG QUESTIONS ABOUT ERGOGENICS

Going beyond genetic endowment and optimal physiological, psychological, and biomechanical training to enhance inherited sports performance factors, many athletes resort to sports ergogenics in attempts to enhance performance and gain competitive edges over their opponents. Surveys reveal that athletes believe ergogenics are an essential component for sport success.

Opinion: "Three out of four track and field athletes competing in Atlanta are using some sort of performance-enhancing drugs."

— *Michael Turner, British Olympic Association Medical Committee*

Surveys also reveal that athletes use a variety of sports ergogenics. Athletes throughout history have used literally hundreds of different nutritional, pharmacological, and physiological sports ergogenics. During the past half-century, the use of sports ergogenics by athletes at all levels of competition appears to have become more prevalent. Several interrelated factors may have contributed to this increase, including (a) the phenomenal increase in the popularity of sports, both professional and amateur, (b) the parallel increase in financial and other benefits accruing to successful athletes, (c) the increasingly sophisticated biomedical and nutritional technological advances leading to the development of drugs and dietary supplements that theoretically may enhance sports performance, and (d) the emergence of sport and exercise science as a respected scientific discipline, with increasing focus on understanding the physiological, psychological, and biomechanical factors underlying successful sport performance, and how such factors might be enhanced.

Looking at considerations other than cost and availability, the answers to four questions might influence your decision to use a specific sports ergogenic in an attempt to enhance performance:

- Is it effective?
- Is it safe?
- Is it legal?
- Is it ethical?

EFFECTIVENESS OF SPORTS ERGOGENICS

It is unlikely that you would use a sports ergogenic unless it worked. But how do you know whether or not a specific sports ergogenic will enhance your performance? You may use several lines of evidence to evaluate its effectiveness, that is, whether it provides the desired effects or results.

Advertisements

As long as athletes believe a magical compound will improve performance, entrepreneurs will market products designed to capitalize on these beliefs. In 12 magazines marketed primarily to bodybuilders, a recent survey of the advertised benefits of nutritional supplements reported 89 brands, 311 products, and 235 unique ingredients; the most frequently promoted supplement and benefit were, respectively, unspecified amino acids and muscle growth.

Companies that manufacture sports ergogenics are in business to make a profit. To further this objective, the truth about a product, particularly nutritional sports ergogenics, might be stretched. For example, amino acids are involved in a variety of important metabolic processes in the human body, including formation of protein to support muscle growth. Thus, an amino acid mixture advertised to "support muscle growth" is acceptable. Although high-quality amino acid supplements can be effective in supporting muscle protein growth, they are considerably more expensive than an equivalent amount of high-quality protein and amino acids obtainable from such natural sources as skim milk or low-fat meat, fish, or poultry.

Advertising can be deceptive and biased in a variety of ways. Research findings taken out of context, endorsement by professional sport organizations, and patented products represent a few deceptive techniques used to advertise purported sports ergogenics; none ensures the product's effectiveness. A patent, for example, indicates only that the product is unique; the U. S. Patent Office does not test its effectiveness.

Articles in Sports Journals and Trade Publications

If you read certain sports magazines, you might get the impression that certain nutritional compounds are essential to optimal performance. Several magazines for bodybuilders frequently contain articles detailing the benefits of amino acid supplements for increasing muscle mass and strength. The publishers of these journals market a variety of expensive amino acid supplements and advertise them extensively in the same journals. The author of the article is protected by the First Amendment, and thus may express the opinion that these supplements may significantly improve muscle growth and strength. On the other hand, advertisements are regulated by the Federal Trade Commission and may not contain any unproven claims. As an astute observer, you should be able to understand why the publisher would print the article and the advertisement in close proximity to each other. As the saying goes, don't believe everything you read. The author might be biased.

In the United States, recently passed legislation (Dietary Supplement Health and Education Act) may exempt dietary supplements from labeling laws. Although the label may not contain scientifically unsupported claims, information materials in the form of an abstract, article, or book chapter may be used in connection with the sale of the dietary supplement to consumers. One of the stipulations is that the information in the materials may not be false or misleading, but the burden of proof is on the Food and Drug Administration (FDA) to demonstrate that the materials violate the law.

In another advertisement technique, some companies put claims of improved physical performance on their product labels, but indicate that these claims have not been evaluated by the FDA. This is a devious way to suggest that these products may be effective sports ergogenics without violating regulations regarding false advertising.

Personal Testimony and Anecdotal Reports

Some companies market their products by using star athletes, whose personal testimony about the product's effectiveness also might be covered by the First Amendment. Examples of this can be found in popular sport magazines. The athlete might not state that the product improves his or her performance, but the impression usually conveyed is that it does. In most cases, the athlete may receive substantial monetary or other benefits to use and/or endorse the product.

A star athlete's use of a purported sports ergogenic does not mean it is effective. The athlete may present a biased viewpoint because of financial rewards.

Personal Experiences

Suppose you see an advertisement for a sports ergogenic endorsed by a star athlete in your sport, so you buy it, try it, and find that it appears to make you feel better in training or competition. Your personal experience may convince you that it is effective. You might, however, be experiencing the placebo effect.

A *placebo* is an inactive substance. Placebos often are used in medicine when patients demand a prescription yet have no physical disease that requires medication. Physicians recognize that many illnesses are psychosomatic, and might prescribe harmless placebos that provide potentially powerful psychological effects. These agents often are effective in curing the patient's problem, i.e., the placebo effect.

A sports ergogenic may work for you not because of any bona fide physiological or mechanical advantage it provides, but because you believe in it, which may benefit you psychologically. Belief in the "magic" of a pill might produce a placebo effect.

On the other hand, sports ergogenics may enhance performance as intended if their effectiveness is supported by appropriate scientific research.

Research Considerations

How do you know whether a particular sports ergogenic will help you improve your sports performance? Deceptive advertisements, biased articles, prejudiced personal testimony, and a placebo effect do not provide sound evidence that a sports ergogenic is effective. Appropriate research is needed to validate the effectiveness of alleged sports ergogenics.

Sport scientists have conducted research on many sports ergogenics, and have made available scientific data for evaluation of their effectiveness. In general, but not always, sport scientists have no financial interest in a specific sports ergogenic; thus, they can provide an unbiased evaluation of its ability to improve performance.

Research findings regarding the effectiveness of specific sports ergogenics are summarized in chapter 8. The recommendations offered regarding the use of each sports ergogenic are based primarily on effectiveness as determined by interpretation of the available well-designed research and research reviews, as well as its safety, legality, and ethicality.

Conducting research to determine the effectiveness of sports ergogenics is not an easy task. In each study, numerous factors must be controlled to ensure valid results. We will not spend a lot of time discussing how to design the perfect study to evaluate the effectiveness of sports ergogenics, but the following considerations are essential for validating the effectiveness of specific sports ergogenics.

Blood doping, a sport physiological ergogenic, is discussed in chapter 8, but will be used here to briefly illustrate research considerations.

1. *Rationale.*   A legitimate rationale must exist. Theoretically, the sports ergogenic should be able to influence favorably a specific sports performance factor (SPF) to enhance either physical power, mental strength, or mechanical edge.

Blood doping may increase hemoglobin levels in the blood to facilitate the transport of oxygen.

2. *Subjects.*   An appropriate subject population should be studied. Subjects should be highly trained in the SPFs that theoretically are enhanced by use of the sports ergogenic. If the sports ergogenic is effective, it should improve performance beyond the effects of training.

Highly trained aerobic endurance athletes, such as marathon runners or road cyclists, should serve as subjects. Blood doping is designed to enhance the oxygen energy system, important to aerobic endurance. See figure 7.1.

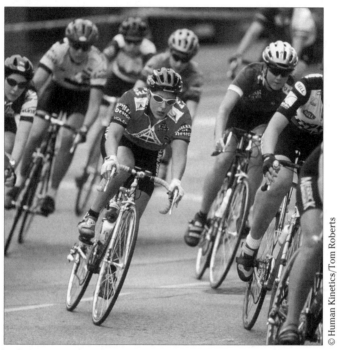

© Human Kinetics/Tom Roberts

Figure 7.1 Subjects involved in studies evaluating the efficacy of sports ergogenics should be well-trained athletes.

3. *Tests.* The tests used to evaluate the SPFs should be valid and reliable. Both laboratory and field tests provide valuable information. Laboratory tests can be well controlled, but do not reflect real-world conditions. Field tests may approach real-world conditions in the athletic arena, but cannot be as well controlled as laboratory tests. Additionally, tests should be conducted to evaluate effects on the underlying rationale for using the sports ergogenic.

A treadmill maximal oxygen uptake ($\dot{V}O_2max$) test and a 10-kilometer road race would represent, respectively, appropriate laboratory and field tests for blood doping (figure 7.2). A blood test for hemoglobin increases would support the underlying rationale.

4. *Learning trials.* Even though well trained, subjects should undertake a learning trial or trials to become proficient in the tests.

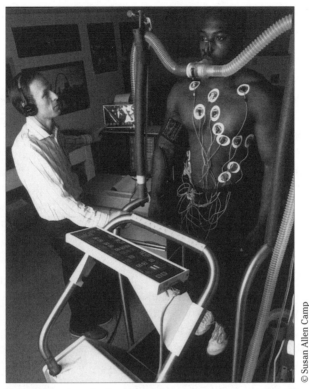

Figure 7.2 Valid laboratory tests should be used to evaluate the efficacy of purported sports ergogenics.

Subjects should learn how to perform a treadmill run to exhaustion to determine $\dot{V}O_2$max or should habitually perform 10-kilometer road races.

5. *Experimental treatment and placebo.* The treatment should be based on sound theoretical rationale. An appropriate placebo should be used, if available.

Two units (1 liter) of infused blood will significantly increase hemoglobin concentration. A saline solution or sham venipuncture can serve as a placebo.

6. *Subject groups.* Subjects should be randomly assigned to the treatment or placebo groups. If possible, subjects should be matched based on the specific SPF test or other key factors and randomly assigned. Although not always feasible, the best design involves a repeated-measures, crossover approach in which each subject randomly takes both the treatment and placebo, with an appropriate washout period between.

Based on preliminary tests, aerobic endurance athletes are matched on maximal oxygen uptake or 10-kilometer road race time and randomly assigned to the treatment or placebo group. With repeated measures, half of the subjects receive the blood infusion and half receive the placebo in the first phase; after a 6-week washout period, the treatment and placebo conditions are switched (crossover) in the second phase.

7. *Double-blind protocol.* Neither the subjects nor the investigators should know which group receives the treatment and which receives the placebo. A third party administers the treatment and placebo and reveals the code at the completion of the study.

Impartial health professionals not involved in the data-collection phase of the study infuse either blood or placebo into the subjects under blinded conditions; the investigators are not informed until completion of the study.

8. *Control of extraneous factors.* Investigators attempt to control extraneous factors that might influence test performance.

During the conduct of the study, the endurance athletes should maintain normal dietary and exercise-training habits. They should prepare for the tests, such as the VO_2max test on the treadmill or 10-kilometer road race, as if preparing for competition.

9. *Control of the testing environment.* The laboratory should be controlled for temperature, humidity, and other factors that might affect the performance test. Field performance tests are not as well controlled, but attempts should be made to duplicate field conditions for each trial.

To field test blood doping, running a competitive 10-kilometer race on an indoor track would help control temperature and wind conditions.

10. *Appropriate statistics.* Appropriate statistical techniques should be used to minimize the chance of statistical error.

An adequate number of subjects and trials should be used. A repeated-measures design increases statistical power because each subject serves as his or her own control.

Evaluation of Available Scientific Research

The most reputable scientific data relative to the effectiveness of purported sports ergogenics appears in peer-reviewed (reviewed by several other experts) scientific journals. The three most common sources of data are: (a) individual studies, (b) reviews by experts, and (c) meta-analyses by appropriate statisticians. The use of sodium bicarbonate supplementation as a sports ergogenic is discussed in chapter 8, but is used here to illustrate these three sources of data.

Individual Studies. Individual studies provide the principal data points, but a single study does not provide conclusive evidence that a sports ergogenic is either effective or ineffective for its stated purpose.

Dozens of studies have been conducted to investigate the ergogenic effect of sodium bicarbonate supplementation. Nearly half of the studies indicated that sodium bicarbonate did not improve sports performance. If you selected one of those studies, you might conclude that sodium bicarbonate was not an effective sports ergogenic. On the other hand, about half of the studies indicate that sodium bicarbonate supplementation improved physical performance.

Headline: Baking soda has no effect on 400-meter dash time.
Headline 6 months later: Baking soda improves 400-meter dash time by 1 second.

Reviews. The effectiveness of sports ergogenics should be supported by a number of well-controlled research studies. A review of previously published individual studies provides a stronger foundation to support effectiveness, but the conclusion may be influenced by the studies reviewed or the reviewer's orientation.

Although reviews some 20 years ago suggested sodium bicarbonate supplementation was not an effective ergogenic, four contemporary reviews concluded that sodium bicarbonate could improve performance in SPFs dependent on the lactic acid energy system.

Meta-Analyses. Meta-analysis of an adequate number of previously published individual studies provides the strongest evidence to support effectiveness. Only well-controlled studies are selected. A *meta-analysis* is a review that provides a summary statistic derived from statistical analyses of all the included studies. In essence, it quantifies the effect of the sports ergogenic.

Twenty-nine well-controlled studies on sodium bicarbonate supplementation were reviewed in a recent meta-analysis. The authors concluded that sodium bicarbonate was a very effective sports ergogenic, increasing by nearly 27 percent sport or exercise performances dependent on the lactic acid energy system.

SAFETY

Safety is an important factor that should influence your decision to use a specific sports ergogenic. Most of the sports ergogenics discussed in chapter 8 can cause adverse health effects in the human body if taken in excessive amounts or used improperly. Although the adverse effects of some sports ergogenics may be acute, mild, and temporary, use of others may elicit chronic, serious, and even life-threatening consequences.

One of the fundamental laws of biology is that any substance that affects living matter may be toxic if taken in excess.

Pharmacological and physiological sports ergogenics pose the most significant health risks. Athletes may use drugs for medicinal, social, or ergogenic purposes. As documented for some specific sports ergogenics in chapter 8, the abuse of drugs for any of these purposes can have serious health consequences.

Nutritional sports ergogenics, ranging from basic nutrients such as vitamins to exotic dietary supplements such as ginseng, are considered safer than pharmacologic sports ergogenics. In general, this may be true. Many nutrients consumed in excess, however, including some vitamins, can impair health. Moreover, some constraints in the United States Dietary Supplement Health and Education Act of 1994 limit the Food and Drug Administration's ability to regulate the safety of dietary supplements. Although some scientists believe dietary supplements are safe, others contend that the safety of some is not substantiated by existing scientific evidence.

You would think that athletes would not intentionally use a sports ergogenic that would impair their health. For some athletes, however, the opportunity for sport success may outweigh any possible health risks, as indicated in the accompanying sidebar.

Unfortunately, little research is available for evaluating the safety of most sports ergogenics. Although the adverse health effects of ergogenic drugs may have received the most research attention, we have very few scientific data regarding adverse health effects associated with chronic supplementation of many dietary supplements and other legal sports ergogenics. Most safety concerns associated with purported sports ergogenics usually are based on in vitro research,

Dr. Robert Voy, a former physician for the United States Olympic Committee and author of *Drugs, Sports, and Politics,* noted that although athletes work hard to make their bodies strong and healthy, they are willing to take serious health risks to gain a competitive edge by using chemical shortcuts. Voy cited an informal study wherein more than 50 percent of elite-level athletes surveyed indicated they would be willing to take a substance that would guarantee them an Olympic gold medal, even if they knew that taking the substance would be fatal within a year.

animal research, or case studies involving people who may have experienced adverse reactions following consumption of a particular product. Although such data might not be the most desirable scientific evidence for evaluating the safety of sports ergogenics in healthy athletes, most sport health professionals seem to believe it wise to err on the side of caution and point out any potential acute or chronic health risks associated with a particular sports ergogenic.

LEGAL STATUS

Another factor that should influence your decision to use a specific sports ergogenic is its legality. All athletic governing bodies have some form of legislation restricting the use of sports ergogenics, so you should be aware of the rules pertaining to your sport.

The use of pharmacological sports ergogenics, or doping, has raised the most concern among the governing bodies.

Anti-doping legislation may have developed out of concern for the health of competing athletes, but the underlying cause of drug use by athletes was performance enhancement. Thus, anti-doping legislation has been designed to prevent cheating and to protect the athlete's health by banning performance-enhancing agents.

The IOC has defined doping as the administration of or the use by a competing athlete of any substance foreign to the body, or of any physiological substance taken in abnormal quantity or by an abnormal route of entry into the body, with the intention of increasing in an artificial and unfair manner his or her performance in competition. Additionally, the IOC indicates that medical treatment with any substance that, because of its nature, dosage, or application, boosts the athlete's performance in competition in an artificial and unfair manner, also is regarded as doping.

The major purpose of this general rule was to discourage the use of drugs by athletes. With some exceptions and limitations noted in chapter 8, most drugs used to enhance performance are prohibited by the IOC and their use by athletes is illegal. For use to be prohibited, the specific agent must be listed by the IOC. The IOC has published an extensive list of prohibited drugs and other sports ergogenics such as blood doping. Some, but not all, of these agents are covered in chapter 8; a detailed list of agents prohibited by the IOC and USOC, and hence by many other sport governing bodies, can be found in appendix A.

In order to enforce anti-doping legislation, a highly technical and effective drug-testing system is available to most athletic governing

> The major purposes of drug testing are to prevent cheating, to protect the health of the athlete, and to promote the integrity of sport.
> — Andrew Pipe, MD, Canadian sport physician

organizations. You most likely would not take illegal drugs in an attempt to improve your sports performance. However, like many athletes, you might take drugs for a variety of medicinal purposes, such as a headache, a stuffed nose, a cold, or to heal an injury. Many over-the-counter medications for such conditions contain drugs prohibited for athletic competition (see figure 7.3). Examples include Sudafed, Dristan, Sinex, and Nyquil (see appendix A). Most athletic governing organizations have brochures or other materials listing prohibited agents and explaining their drug-testing procedures, which may include unannounced drug tests.

If you will be competing in any athletic event involving drug testing, such as a USA Track & Field-sponsored road race or NCAA contest, it would be advisable to check with your athletic governing body about the legality of any medications you are taking.

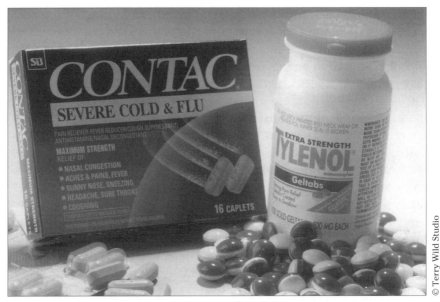

Figure 7.3 Many over-the-counter (OTC) drugs for common illnesses such as colds and headaches contain drugs prohibited by the International Olympic Committee.

ETHICAL ISSUES

What are the ethics of sport? According to the Oxford English Dictionary, the definition for ethics includes the following: (a) moral principles of a particular school of thought, (b) rules of conduct recognized in certain associations, and (c) moral principles by which an individual is guided.

All three definitions are operational in sports. The ancient Greek ideal, that athletes should succeed through their unaided efforts, is a school of thought (definition a) embraced by many athletes and organizations today, including the International Olympic Committee. Within this committee, certain associations, such as the International Amateur Cycling Federation, establish specific rules of conduct (definition b) to promote athletes' adherence to the Greek ideal and to discourage them from obtaining unfair advantages. The athlete whose primary goal is to win at all costs may be guided by his or her own principles (definition c) in an attempt to obtain that unfair advantage.

We have all heard the Olympic ideal paraphrased as "Do the best you can with what you've got." The "what you've got" originally referred to the athlete's natural athletic abilities, finely tuned through vigorous physical training with the guidance of a coach and trainer. An increasing number of elite athletes participating in international competition, however, are learning to modify their natural ability by techniques that go beyond normal training in order to get an advantage—and not necessarily an unfair one—over their competitors. They are assisted in these endeavors by a variety of sport scientists, including sport physicians, sport physiologists, sport nutritionists, sport psychologists, sport biomechanists, and even sport pharmacologists.

The use of sports ergogenics that are specifically prohibited by IOC anti-doping rules, such as anabolic steroids and blood doping, certainly would be considered unethical behavior. An IOC general definition of doping stipulates, however, that any physiological substance taken in abnormal quantity with the intention of artificially and unfairly increasing performance should be construed as doping. Over the past few decades, sport scientists have documented the important roles of various nutrients and physiological substances on energy metabolism during exercise. Although all nutrients and physiological substances may be obtained either directly or indirectly through a normal diet, some investigators believe the intake of several nutrients or physiological substances important for energy metabolism may be limited through normal dietary practices. Through modern biotechnology, a wide array of dietary supplements and physiological substances have been isolated and manufactured in quantity. Some of these products purported to be ergogenic, such as human growth hormone, have been grouped with drugs and their use has been prohibited by the IOC. Use of other products, such as specific amino acids theorized to stimulate the natural formation of human growth hormone, has not been prohibited presumably because they may be classified as nutrients.

An athlete's use of pharmacological and physiological ergogenics may be grounds for suspension from sports competition, so considerable research has been conducted in attempts to find effective, safe, and legal nutritional ergogenics. No nutritional or physiological dietary supplement is prohibited unless the supplement contains an illegal substance. The stimulant ephedrine, for example, is found in several commercial dietary supplements. Some current research suggests that several physiological sports ergogenics, such as creatine, might enhance specific SPFs when consumed in amounts much greater than would be consumed in a normal diet. If physiological and nutritional sports ergogenics are shown to be effective, do they violate the IOC general doping rule regarding any physiological substance taken in abnormal quantity with the intention of artificially and unfairly increasing performance?

According to the IOC, use of an alleged sports ergogenic is prohibited only if it is specifically named, which seems to be at odds with the general doping rule relative to positive ergogenic effects resulting from any substance taken in abnormal amounts. This stipulation of the IOC might be a cause of ethical concern for some athletes, and possibly could put them at a competitive disadvantage if they do not use effective, legal sports ergogenics while their competitors do.

As noted in chapter 8, effective, safe, and legal ergogenics are available. Whether their use is ethical may depend on the individual athlete's code of ethics. Some authorities may consider that because a sports ergogenic is legal, its use is ethical. Others may contend that such a sports ergogenic violates the ethics of the IOC anti-doping rule. In this situation, the ultimate decision about whether to use a legal, safe, and effective sports ergogenic rests with the individual athlete.

RECOMMENDATIONS AND INDIVIDUALITY

Results reported in scientific journals usually focus on the effect of a sports ergogenic on a group of individuals. Although all humans share similar anatomical and physiological traits, we possess biological individuality due either to basic hereditary differences or environmental modifications. For example, the responses you have to sodium bicarbonate prior to a competitive event might vary. Although research supports the effectiveness of sodium bicarbonate as a sports ergogenic, its use might be detrimental to some people. Conversely, although research may not support the effectiveness of other purported sports ergogenics, you might benefit from their use. Although vitamin supplementation, in general, has little support as an effective sports ergogenic, you might benefit if you participate in a weight-control sport and are on a very-low-calorie diet to make weight, and thus might have a marginal vitamin intake that could be remedied by an appropriate supplement.

The recommendations provided in chapter 8 relative to the use of each specific sports ergogenic are grounded not only on research-based effectiveness, but also on safety, legal issues, and ethical concerns.

RATING THE SPORTS ERGOGENICS

Athletes consume or use hundreds of different sports ergogenics in attempts to enhance physical power, mental strength, or mechanical edge. Most of those that have been used and studied to determine their effectiveness will be discussed in this chapter.

Each sports ergogenic will be discussed according to the following format:

Classification and Usage

What is it and how is it used? A sports ergogenic may be classified as either nutritional, pharmacological, or physiological. Common names, types, sources, and normal usage procedures, if available, will be identified. Amounts used in research normally are presented in metric units. A brief conversion table for international (metric) and English units is presented in appendix B.

Sports Performance Factor

Which athletes might benefit from its use? A sports ergogenic may be designed to influence one or more SPFs related to physical power, mental strength, or mechanical edge. Chapter 6 provides a brief review of these factors. For an extended discussion, see chapters 3, 4, and 5.

Theory

How is it supposed to work? A sports ergogenic should have a sound theoretical basis underlying its alleged effect on sports performance. The logic underlying the theory will be examined.

Effectiveness

Does it work? The ability of a sports ergogenic to enhance physical performance should be supported by well-controlled experimental research, preferably including both laboratory and field studies. Available contemporary research findings will be summarized. You may wish to review the section on the use of research to determine effectiveness in chapter 7.

Safety

Is it safe to use? Used properly, a sports ergogenic should be harmless. Possible acute and chronic health risks will be addressed. You may wish to review the section on safety in chapter 7.

Legal Aspects and Ethical Issues

Is its use legal and ethical? Athletics governing bodies, such as the International Olympic Committee and National Collegiate Athletic Association, have prohibited most effective pharmacological and physiological sports ergogenics; thus their use may be regarded as both illegal and unethical. Some effective, legal sports ergogenics have not been prohibited, but some may consider their use to be unethical. These points will be noted. You may wish to review the section on legal status and ethical issues in chapter 7.

Recommendations

Should you use it? In general, a sports ergogenic may be recommended if its use is effective, safe, legal, and ethical. Conversely, a sports ergogenic will not be recommended if its use is either ineffective or detrimental, unsafe, illegal, or unethical. A general recommendation for each sports ergogenic will be made, but may be qualified in relation to potential chronic health risks or questions of ethicality. One caveat: If you plan to use any sports ergogenic in conjunction with competition, experiment with it in training first.

USING THIS CHAPTER

If you are interested in sports ergogenics that might influence performance in your sport, follow this three-step procedure.

1. From table 6.2 (pages 85–92), list the sports performance factor or factors (SPFs) that are intrinsic to your sport. If your specific sport is not listed, find one that is comparable.
2. From table 6.3 (pages 94–97), list the sports ergogenics that have been studied in attempts to improve the SPFs for your sport.
3. In this chapter, review the information regarding each specific sports ergogenic in order to make a decision regarding its suitability for use.

Alcohol

Classification and Usage

Alcohol may be classified as a pharmacological sports ergogenic. Alcohol (ethyl alcohol, ethanol) is a social drug classified as a depressant, although its use can elicit a paradoxical stimulant effect. Alcohol is derived from the fermentation of sugars in fruits, vegetables, and grains and contains caloric energy, approximately 7 calories per gram. One drink of alcohol, the equivalent of one bottle of beer, 4–5 ounces of wine, and 1.25 ounces of standard bar liquor, contains about 14 grams of alcohol (figure 8.1). Athletes who might benefit from alcohol consume it 30–60 minutes prior to competition.

Sports Performance Factor

Mental strength. Alcohol has been studied primarily in attempts to decrease the adverse effects of psychological stress during precision sports such as archery, riflery, and dart throwing. Because alcohol use is prevalent in society, its effects on physical power have been studied.

Theory

Through its depressant activity on the nervous system, alcohol might enhance precision sports performance by reducing the adverse effects of anxiety on motor control, particularly by reducing hand tremors. Some investigators contend that alcohol may increase self-confidence, which could improve performance in a variety of sports.

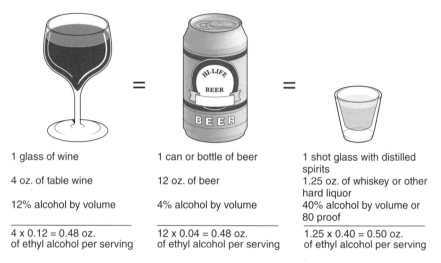

1 glass of wine	1 can or bottle of beer	1 shot glass with distilled spirits
4 oz. of table wine	12 oz. of beer	1.25 oz. of whiskey or other hard liquor
12% alcohol by volume	4% alcohol by volume	40% alcohol by volume or 80 proof
4 x 0.12 = 0.48 oz. of ethyl alcohol per serving	12 x 0.04 = 0.48 oz. of ethyl alcohol per serving	1.25 x 0.40 = 0.50 oz. of ethyl alcohol per serving

Figure 8.1 A 12-ounce bottle of beer, a 4-ounce glass of wine, and 1.25 ounces of bar whiskey contain about the same amount of alcohol.

It has been theorized that alcohol is a source of energy during aerobic endurance exercise.

Effectiveness

Although it may be theorized that alcohol improves performance by reducing anxiety or hand tremor, only a few studies have investigated the effect of alcohol on precision sports performance. In a well-controlled study with archers, alcohol exerted some contrasting effects. Small doses of alcohol resulted in slower reaction times and a decrease in hand steadiness—factors that would impair performance. The use of alcohol also resulted in a smoother release of the arrow, which would improve performance. Unfortunately, no actual performance data were reported. In another study, dart-throwing accuracy improved at a *blood alcohol concentration* (BAC) of 0.02, the equivalent of one drink, but was impaired at a BAC of 0.05, about two drinks.

Use of alcohol may actually impair performance in other sports. Research overwhelmingly supports the conclusion that alcohol adversely affects performance in perceptual-motor sports—those involving skills such as reaction time, balance, hand/eye coordination, and visual perception—such as tennis.

Additionally, alcohol consumption may impair performance in

anaerobic and aerobic endurance performance; alcohol exerted a detrimental effect in both an 800-meter and 1,500-meter run, the effect being dose-related as adverse effects increased with increasing BACs from .01 to .10.

For athletes who drink socially, research has indicated that alcohol consumption in moderation (1–2 drinks) does not impair sports performance factors the following day. Excess consumption to the extent of intoxication, however, has been shown to impair perceptual motor and aerobic endurance performance the following day, and chronic excessive alcohol intake might impair training and, subsequently, performance.

Safety

Consumed in moderation as a social drug, alcohol is safe and might confer some health benefits, such as reduction of coronary artery disease. Conversely, excess acute alcohol consumption is a major risk factor for accidental death, while excess chronic consumption is associated with pathological conditions including liver damage, heart disease, and cancer.

Legal and Ethical Aspects

The use of alcohol in conjunction with competition is formally prohibited only for modern pentathlon, which includes shooting events. Testing for alcohol may be requested by any *national governing body* (NGB) and a positive test could lead to sanctions. Sanctions are most likely for athletes in the 11 pistol and 2 archery events in Olympic competition, as well as in other sports in which excess anxiety might interfere with performance, such as figure skating, ski jumping, diving, fencing, gymnastics, and synchronized swimming. The use of alcohol in conjunction with these sports would be unethical.

Recommendations

Although research is limited but tends to support the ergogenic effectiveness of alcohol use in precision sports such as archery and dart throwing, its use is illegal in conjunction with these sports and cannot be recommended. Alcohol use is not prohibited for other sports. As noted, however, when consumed in conjunction with competition or in excess during training or on the evening before competition, the use of alcohol might impair performance in a variety of other sports.

Amphetamines

Classification and Usage

Amphetamines may be classified as a pharmacological sports ergogenic. Amphetamines are prescription drugs that have been used therapeutically in the treatment of narcolepsy (a sleeping disorder), attention deficit disorder (hyperactivity) in children, and as an appetite depressant.

Although amphetamines have bona fide medical applications, they also are popular recreational drugs. Amphetamines such as Benzedrine and Dexedrine (bennies, uppers, pep pills) were readily available in the 1950s and 1960s until their use was controlled by legislation. Other derivatives of amphetamine, including methamphetamine (meth, speed) and methylenedioxymethamphetamine (MDMA, ecstasy), are used recreationally for their mood-altering effects. Amphetamines come in tablet or powder form and are swallowed, inhaled, or injected (figure 8.2). Benzedrine and Dexedrine were most commonly used in research, with doses approximating 5–15 milligrams.

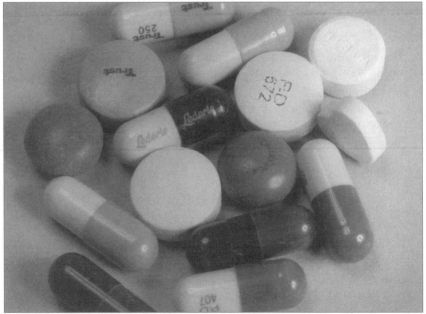

© Terry Wild Studio

Figure 8.2 Amphetamines are powerful stimulants that may influence a variety of sports performance factors.

Sports Performance Factor

Mental strength, physical power, and mechanical edge. Amphetamines have been studied in attempts to enhance various sports performance factors that might benefit from a supplemental mental stimulant effect, including the effects on physical power derived from all three human energy systems—the ATP-CP, lactic acid, and oxygen energy systems—as well as from improved mechanical edge through loss of body fat.

Theory

Amphetamines are powerful central nervous system (CNS) stimulants that act primarily by enhancing the brain activity of norepinephrine and dopamine, intensifying psychological sensations of alertness, arousal, concentration, and self-confidence. Physiologic responses associated with amphetamine-induced CNS stimulation include increased muscle contractility, increased blood flow to the muscle, and a decreased sense of fatigue. In general, it has been theorized that the psychological effects of amphetamines permit athletes to go beyond their normal physiologic limits. Amphetamines also are powerful appetite-suppressant drugs.

Effectiveness

Amphetamines appear to be a potent sports ergogenic. Although not all studies show positive results, research supports the findings that amphetamine use might improve reaction time when fatigued, increase muscular strength and endurance, increase acceleration, increase lactic acid levels at maximal exercise, and increase aerobic endurance capacity. Research also shows that amphetamines might decrease the appetite and stimulate metabolism, inducing a loss of body fat.

Safety

Reported adverse side effects of recreational amphetamine use include headaches, dizziness, sleeplessness, and anxiety. Use of higher doses are associated with mental confusion, hallucinations, skin disorders, and ulcers. Heavy use may be associated with brain damage. There is a high rate of morbidity and mortality among children born to women who abuse amphetamines. Use of needles to inject amphetamines increases the risk for hepatitis and AIDS.

Amphetamine use may carry significant health risks for the athlete, as evidenced by several amphetamine-linked deaths in sport.

Amphetamines may interfere with temperature regulation, leading to hyperthermia during exercise. The death of a Danish cyclist in the 1960 Rome Olympics and other amphetamine-related sport tragedies served as catalysts for the development of anti-doping legislation by the International Olympic Committee.

The purity of street amphetamine products may vary. These look-alikes contain less potent stimulants, such as caffeine and ephedrine, encouraging consumption of larger doses to get an effect similar to that of amphetamines. If an individual buys pure amphetamine but thinks it is a look-alike and consumes more, the results could be toxic.

Legal and Ethical Aspects

Amphetamine use is prohibited by most athletic governing bodies and is considered unethical behavior. Drug testing has been effective in detecting amphetamine metabolites in the urine of athletes. Comparable to amphetamines, use by athletes of numerous related stimulants and even over-the-counter medications (decongestants and cold medications) containing stimulants has been prohibited by the IOC. A partial list may be found in appendix A. Additionally, amphetamines are a controlled drug and illegal distribution or use may be subject to criminal penalties.

Recommendations

Research supports the ergogenic effectiveness of amphetamines. Amphetamine use is not recommended, however, because it is illegal, unethical, and might significantly increase health risks in some athletes.

Anabolic Phytosterols (Plant Sterols)

Classification and Usage

Phytosterols, or plant sterols, are dietary supplements that may be classified as a nutritional sports ergogenic. They are extracted from various plants and vegetables. Several phytosterols and their derivatives are marketed to strength-trained athletes; common types include gamma oryzanol, Smilax, beta-sitosterol, and ferulic acid. Other plant extracts, such as ginseng and yohimbine, also are marketed to athletes.

Anabolic phytosterols are sold separately or in combination with other purported nutritional sports ergogenics. Recommended dosages vary depending on the product.

Sports Performance Factor

Mechanical edge and physical power. Anabolic phytochemicals are used primarily to increase muscle mass and decrease body fat for enhanced strength and power, or for a more aesthetic physical appearance in sports such as bodybuilding.

Theory

Anabolic phytosterols are advertised as a means of stimulating the release of testosterone or human growth hormone, both anabolic hormones that can increase muscle mass and decrease body fat.

Effectiveness

Several recent reviews concluded that there is no scientific evidence that any so-called anabolic phytosterol increases the release of testosterone or human growth hormone, much less leads to an increase in muscle mass and decrease in body fat. Human studies are almost nonexistent, and, based on metabolic findings in animal studies, one reviewer indicates that gamma oryzanol supplementation might suppress testosterone secretion.

Safety

Many herbal products, including phytosterols, lack appropriate safety data. It has been reported that some preparations cause health problems, and fatalities from anaphylactic reactions have been reported.

Legal and Ethical Aspects

Supplementation with purported anabolic phytochemicals as a sports ergogenic is both legal and ethical.

Recommendations

Supplementation with purported anabolic phytochemicals is not recommended as a sports ergogenic because no reputable scientific data support their effectiveness to enhance performance. Moreover, their use may be associated with adverse health effects.

Anabolic/Androgenic Steroids (AAS)

Classification and Usage

Anabolic/androgenic steroids (AAS) may be classified as a pharmacological sports ergogenic. AAS are prescription drugs designed to mimic the effects of testosterone, the natural male sex hormone. Anabolic effects of testosterone include growth and development of many body tissues, including muscle tissue. Androgenic effects include the development of male secondary sex characteristics, such as facial hair.

AAS are available for oral consumption or injection. A few of the more popular anabolic steroids are listed in table 8.1; a more complete list is found in appendix A. AAS have beneficial medical applications, a normal therapeutic dose being about 5 to 10 milligrams per day for the oral compounds. It has been reported that many athletes take up to 300 milligrams and more daily. Some athletes practice a technique called *stacking*, which involves the use of two or more steroids at a time, usually both oral and injectable AAS. Stacking might also involve a progressive increase in the types and dosages of AAS in order to obtain an optimal anabolic effect. Athletes might take other drugs to prevent some of the undesirable effects of AAS. For example, human chorionic gonadotropin might prevent atrophy of the testicles and antiestrogens might prevent development of female-like breast appearance in males. The use of two or more drugs at one time has been characterized as the *polydrug abuse syndrome*.

TABLE 8.1
Trade and Generic Names for Commonly Used
Anabolic/Androgenic Steroids

Oral compounds
Anadrol (oxymetholone)
Anavar (oxandrolone)
Dianabol (methandrostenolone)
Metandren (methyltestosterone)
Primobolin (methenolone)
Winstrol (stanozolol)

Injectable compounds
Deca-durabolin (nandrolone decanoate)
Delatestryl (testosterone enanthate)
Depo-testosterone (testosterone cypionate)
Testosterone suspension

Sports Performance Factor

Mechanical edge and physical power. AAS have been studied primarily in attempts to increase muscle mass for enhanced strength and power or for a more aesthetic physical appearance in sports such as bodybuilding; AAS may also affect mental processes, increasing aggressive behavior.

Theory

The use of AAS may influence both physiological and psychological processes associated with enhanced sports performance. The anabolic mechanism of AAS is depicted in figure 8.3. The AAS influence the cell nucleus to enhance muscle protein formation. AAS also might help prevent the breakdown of muscle tissue, possibly leading to a more rapid recovery from intense training. Additionally, androgenic effects of AAS may include increased arousal and aggressiveness in some individuals, psychological effects which have been suggested to help athletes train and perform more intensely. Although AAS are used extensively by strength/power athletes, endurance athletes also might benefit from enhanced recovery that would permit more intense training.

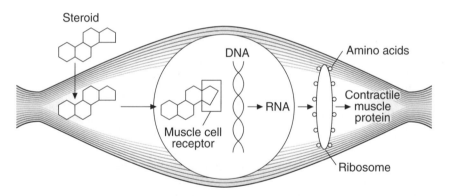

Figure 8.3 Anabolic steroids picked up by receptors in the cell nucleus initiate the process of protein formation in cells such as muscle fibers.

Effectiveness

Dozens of studies have been conducted to evaluate the ergogenic effectiveness of AAS. These studies have been the subject of several detailed reviews, most notably by the American College of Sport

Medicine and Dr. Janet Elashoff, the latter review involving a partial meta-analysis. Although these reviewers noted that the research findings are somewhat equivocal because of differences in experimental design, they concluded that the use of AAS in conjunction with an appropriate resistance-training program and diet will increase lean muscle mass and strength. In laboratory studies, the AAS dosages used were normally minimal, about 5–10 milligrams, and hence the lean muscle mass and strength gains were smaller. However, case studies with strength/power athletes who used higher dosages and stacking techniques, but who cycled on and off AAS, have provided evidence of potent gains in both lean muscle mass and strength during the on cycle.

AAS are effective as a pharmacological sports ergogenic to increase muscle mass and strength. The effects of AAS on actual sport performance have not been studied extensively, but one might assume that the reported benefits on muscle mass and strength would lead to improvements in sports tasks dependent on explosive strength and power.

Safety

AAS are potent drugs; their use might elicit adverse effects ranging from changes in cosmetic appearance, such as acne, to life-threatening disorders, such as heart disease. Additionally, black-market sources of AAS might contain preparations of unknown quality and composition that could increase health risks, as can the use of other drugs in polydrug abuse. AAS can upset normal hormonal balance by interfering with the normal feedback control between the hypothalamus, pituitary gland, and the gonads. AAS, particularly oral compounds, are catabolized in the liver and might impair normal liver function. AAS also might increase aggressive behavior, perhaps contributing to abnormal behavior and associated health risks. Table 8.2 highlights some of the health risks associated with the use of AAS.

Legal and Ethical Aspects

AAS are one of the most abused drugs in sports competition. AAS use is prohibited by most athletic governing bodies and is considered unethical behavior. Drug testing has been effective in detection of AAS metabolites in the urine of athletes, and has led to the disqualification of Olympic champions who have admitted to using AAS. Some athletes who testified that they had not consumed AAS tested positive for AAS metabolites. AAS is injected into the muscle of animals, such as

TABLE 8.2
Possible Health Risks Associated With Use of
Anabolic/Androgenic Steroids

Cosmetic-related effects
Facial and body acne
Female-like breast enlargement in males
Premature baldness
Masculinization in females
Facial and body hair growth in females
Premature closure of growth centers in adolescents, leading to stunted growth
Deepening of the voice in females

Psychologic effects
Increased aggressiveness and possible violent behavior

Reproductive effects
Reduction of testicular size
Reduction of sperm production
Decreased libido
Impotence in males
Enlargement of the prostate gland
Enlargement of the clitoris

Cardiovascular risk factors and diseases
Atherosclerotic serum lipid profile
  Decreased HDL-cholesterol
  Increased LDL-cholesterol
High blood pressure
Impaired glucose tolerance
Stroke
Heart disease

Liver function
Jaundice
Peliosis hepatis (blood-filled cysts)
Liver tumors

Athletic injuries
Tendon rupture

AIDS
Use of contaminated needles

chickens, to promote growth of lean tissue prior to marketing. Recent research revealed positive urine tests for AAS metabolites in athletes who had eaten animal meat that had been injected with AAS.

Illegally distributing AAS on the black market is a criminal offense, punishable by fines and prison terms.

Recommendations

Research supports the ergogenic effectiveness of AAS. However, AAS use is not recommended because it is illegal, unethical, and may significantly increase health risks.

Antioxidants

Classification and Usage

Antioxidants are nutrients or dietary supplements that may be classified as a nutritional sports ergogenic. Although a number of commercial antioxidant products are targeted to athletes, the most common are the vitamins beta-carotene, vitamin C, and vitamin E; the mineral selenium; and the dietary supplement coenzyme Q_{10}. They are marketed singly, in combination, or with other alleged antioxidant substances in an antioxidant cocktail. Some sports bars are fortified with antioxidants.

Dosages of antioxidant cocktails used in research with humans have varied. One study combined 22.5 milligrams of beta-carotene, 750 milligrams of vitamin C, 600 International Units (IU) of vitamin E, and 100 milligrams of coenzyme Q_{10}.

Sports Performance Factor

Physical power. Antioxidant cocktails may be used in attempts to increase all types of physical power from the three human energy systems, the ATP-CP, lactic acid, and oxygen energy systems.

Theory

Strenuous exercise increases the production of oxygen free radicals either during exercise or in the recovery period. To help counteract the damaging peroxidation effects of free radicals on lipid cell membranes and other cellular structures, tissues in the human body produce several antioxidant enzymes (glutathione peroxidase, catalase, superoxide dismutase). It is theorized that antioxidant supplements bolster these natural antioxidant defenses and help prevent

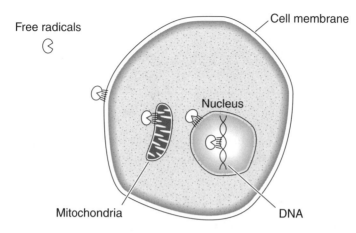

Free radicals

Cell membrane

Nucleus

Mitochondria

DNA

Figure 8.4 Free radicals may damage cell membranes and membranes of intracellular structures, including mitochondria, the nucleus, and DNA.

muscle and other tissue damage during strenuous aerobic endurance training (figure 8.4). By preventing such damage, the athlete may be able to train all human energy systems more effectively and enhance performance in a variety of sports competition.

Effectiveness

Numerous studies have investigated the effect of antioxidant supplements on markers of muscle tissue damage; the results are inconclusive but promising. Scientific experts indicate that although trained individuals may have a greater need for antioxidants, the ability of antioxidant supplements to prevent exercise-induced lipid peroxidation and muscle damage remains to be established.

Safety

Vitamin and mineral antioxidants consumed in amounts no greater than the Recommended Dietary Allowances appear to be safe. Excessive amounts of any antioxidant might elicit toxic side effects.

Legal and Ethical Aspects

Antioxidant supplementation is legal and ethical in conjunction with sport competition.

Recommendations

Based on available scientific evidence, antioxidant supplementation has not been shown to enhance sport performance and has not been validated as an effective sports ergogenic, hence its use is not recommended for this purpose.

Some investigators note that because antioxidant vitamin supplementation may play a protective role against muscle tissue damage during strenuous training, and because their use is relatively harmless, such supplements might be recommended for individuals performing regular heavy exercise.

One scientist recommends that athletes who train intensely consume substantial amounts of beta-carotene (50,000 IU), vitamin C

TABLE 8.3
Good Food Sources and Approximate Amounts of the Antioxidant Vitamins

Beta-carotene

1 medium apricot = 800 International Units

1/2 cup cooked broccoli = 550 International Units

1 cup cantaloupe = 5,000 International Units

1 carrot = 20,000 International Units

1 mango = 8,000 International Units

1 papaya = 6,000 International Units

1/2 cup cooked spinach = 7,000 International Units

1 baked sweet potato = 25,000 International Units

Vitamin C

1/2 cup cooked broccoli = 50 milligrams

4 ounces grapefruit juice = 45 milligrams

1 mango = 55 milligrams

4 ounces orange juice = 60 milligrams

1 papaya = 190 milligrams

1/2 cup strawberries = 40 milligrams

Vitamin E

1 ounce almonds = 8 International Units

1 tablespoon margarine = 8 International Units

1 tablespoon mayonnaise = 10 International Units

1 tablespoon sunflower oil = 6 International Units

1 ounce sunflower seeds = 14 International Units

1/4 cup dry wheat germ = 4 International Units

1 tablespoon wheat germ oil = 20 International Units

(women 2,000 milligrams and men 3,000 milligrams), and vitamin E (1,200 IU). These recommendations are not offered as a way to enhance sports performance, but possibly to prevent adverse health effects, such as cancer, which are associated with excessive oxygen free radical generation. These recommendations are rather substantial and most likely would require the use of supplements because they are unlikely to be obtained from the normal diet.

Most athletes ideally should obtain adequate amounts of the nutrient antioxidants through their diets, selecting foods rich in beta-carotene, vitamin C, and vitamin E, as noted in table 8.3. A healthful diet rich in fruits and vegetables will increase the dietary intake of beta-carotene and vitamin C, while vegetable oils are a good source of vitamin E. Natural foods also may contain other substances, known as phytochemicals, which might be protective against the development of chronic diseases such as cancer.

If you decide to take antioxidant supplements as an adjunct to your intense exercise training regimen, dosages of 500 to 1,000 milligrams of vitamin C, 400 to 800 IU of vitamin E, and 50 to 100 micrograms of selenium may be safe intakes and may help complement your natural antioxidant enzymes, particularly if you do not consume a diet rich in these nutrients.

Vitamins C and E, selenium, and coenzyme Q_{10} have been studied individually for sports ergogenic potential and are discussed elsewhere in this chapter.

Arginine, Lysine, and Ornithine

Classification and Usage

Arginine, lysine, and ornithine may be classified as nutritional sports ergogenics. *Arginine* and *ornithine* are nonessential amino acids, meaning they may be formed in the body from other amino acids; *lysine* is an essential amino acid, meaning it must be obtained in the diet. These amino acids are natural constituents of protein, but they do not exist in free form in foods we eat. The Recommended Dietary Allowance for lysine is somewhat less than 1 gram per day, which is easily obtainable in the typical diet.

Arginine, lysine, and ornithine are available commercially in tablet or powder form either individually or in combination. Typical doses used in research approximated a total of 2–3 grams per day, usually in equal dosages when the amino acids were used in combination.

Sports Performance Factor

Mechanical edge and physical power. Arginine, lysine, and ornithine have been studied primarily in attempts to increase muscle mass and decrease body fat for enhanced strength and power, or for a more aesthetic physical appearance in sports such as bodybuilding. Some products have been marketed as being more effective than anabolic/ androgenic steroids.

Theory

Oral intake of arginine, lysine, or ornithine is theorized to increase circulating levels of several hormones, particularly *human growth hormone (hGH)* and insulin. Thus the proposed ergogenic effect of these amino acids is attributed to the anabolic effects of hGH and insulin. Briefly, it is theorized that hGH and insulin increase muscle mass and decrease body fat.

Effectiveness

Although the infusion of certain amino acids may increase circulating hGH and insulin levels, four contemporary well-controlled studies do not support comparable effects with oral supplementation. These studies, all involving experienced, resistance-trained males, found no effect of oral supplementation with arginine, lysine, or ornithine, or with combinations of other amino acids, on blood hGH or insulin levels. One study from Finland reported that 4 days of supplementation with 2 grams each of arginine, lysine, and ornithine had no effect on circulating levels of either hGH or insulin measured periodically over 24 hours. Another study indicated very high oral doses of ornithine might increase circulating hGH, but not insulin, levels. Unfortunately, these dosages, approximating 10 grams or more, caused gastrointestinal distress, that is, diarrhea.

Several of these studies also evaluated the ergogenic potential of arginine, lysine, or ornithine supplementation with experienced weight lifters, and found no significant effect on body fat, lean muscle mass, or muscular strength, power, and endurance.

Safety

Although no reports of adverse health effects have been reported in studies using up to 6 grams per day, consumption of larger amounts of individual amino acids may cause gastrointestinal distress. Additionally, some health professionals contend that consumption of excess amounts of specific oral amino acid supplements might inhibit the absorption of other amino acids into the body.

Legal and Ethical Aspects

Arginine, lysine, and ornithine supplements are legal. Currently there does not appear to be an ethical problem with their use in conjunction with sports performance.

Recommendations

Resistance-trained athletes may need more protein in their diet when attempting to increase lean muscle mass, but no reputable scientific evidence indicates that arginine, lysine, and ornithine supplementation provides any additional benefit. Supplementation with these amino acids therefore is not recommended for athletes.

Aspartates (Aspartic Acid Salts)

Classification and Usage

Aspartates, salts of aspartic acid, may be classified as a nutritional sports ergogenic. *Aspartic acid* is a nonessential amino acid and a natural constituent of protein, but it does not exist in free form in foods we eat.

Aspartates are available commercially as potassium and magnesium aspartate in tablet or powder form. Daily dosages used in research studies averaged 7 to 10 grams consumed over a 24-hour period.

Sports Performance Factor

Physical power. Aspartates are designed to enhance aerobic power and endurance for sport events that derive energy primarily from the oxygen energy system.

Theory

Although the mechanism underlying the purported ergogenic effect of aspartate supplementation has not been delineated, several hypotheses have been advanced. First, it has been suggested that aspartates increase the use of free fatty acids (FFA) for energy production, which might spare the use of muscle glycogen. Second, aspartates may reduce the accumulation of ammonia in the blood; increases in serum ammonia may cause fatigue, but the mechanism is not known. Theoretically, sparing of muscle glycogen and reduced ammonia accumulation could enhance performance in prolonged aerobic endurance events.

Effectiveness

The research findings regarding the ergogenic effect of aspartate supplementation are inconclusive. Five well-controlled studies, using similar dosages of aspartates (6 to 10 grams of potassium and magnesium aspartate over 24 hours) and exercise endurance testing protocols (treadmill running or cycle ergometer rides to exhaustion at 60 percent to 75 percent of VO_2max) produced divergent results. Two of the studies found that aspartate supplementation exerted no significant effect on physiological or metabolic responses to exercise, such as heart rate, serum lactate levels, and an increased use of FFA for energy, or on exercise time to exhaustion. Conversely, three studies reported significant improvements of 15 percent, 22 percent, and 37 percent in exercise time to exhaustion, with one study finding an increased mobilization of FFA and a decreased accumulation of blood ammonia.

Although additional research is necessary to resolve these differences and to determine underlying mechanisms, potassium and magnesium aspartate supplementation might be effective sports ergogenics. It should be noted, however, that magnesium is theorized to provide an ergogenic effect in aerobic endurance events.

Safety

No adverse side effects have been reported from individuals consuming potassium and magnesium aspartates on a short-term (10 grams in 24 hours) or long-term (8 grams daily for 18 months) basis. Larger doses may cause osmotic diarrhea.

Legal and Ethical Aspects

Aspartates are legal. Currently there does not appear to be an ethical problem with their use in conjunction with sports performance. If they eventually are shown to be effective ergogenics, however, some might consider their use to be unethical.

Recommendations

Supplementation with potassium and magnesium aspartates is legal, safe, apparently ethical, and might be ergogenic, although additional corroborative research is needed.

Carbohydrate is the recommended energy source for the aerobic endurance athlete, so adequate dietary carbohydrate is needed both before and during prolonged aerobic endurance exercise. Adding potassium and magnesium aspartates to the diet should complement, not replace, carbohydrate sources of energy. Although not completely proven, about 10 grams of potassium and magnesium aspartates, consumed in five 2-gram doses over a 24-hour period, would be an acceptable procedure. Experiment with aspartate supplementation in training before using in competition.

Bee Pollen

Classification and Usage

Bee pollen is a dietary supplement that may be classified as a nutritional sports ergogenic. Although the precise chemical analysis is unclear, harvested bee pollen is a mixture of vitamins, minerals, amino acids, and other trace nutrients. Commercial bee pollen is available in capsules. Up to 2.7 grams daily have been used in research with sports performance.

Sports Performance Factor

Physical power. Bee pollen has been advertised as increasing high power, power endurance, and aerobic power, thus affecting all three human energy systems.

Theory

No specific chemical in bee pollen has been identified as being ergogenic, but any benefit is believed to be a collective effect of the multiple nutrients. Advertising claims promote the theory that bee pollen may be a good energy food, particularly designed to facilitate recovery from intense exercise training. Although this theory is based on poorly controlled field research, anecdotal reports of enhanced performance from world-class athletes, ranging from Olympic sprinters to marathoners, have promoted its use.

Effectiveness

There are no reputable published studies supporting an ergogenic effect of bee pollen supplementation. Six well-controlled studies reported that bee pollen supplementation had no effect on metabolic, physiological, and psychological responses to exercise, VO_2max, or endurance capacity in several exercise tasks. One study tested the theory of enhanced recovery with highly trained runners and reported no significant effect of varying doses of bee pollen supplementation on the rate of recovery as measured by performance in repeated maximal treadmill runs to exhaustion with set recovery periods.

Safety

Containing mostly nutrients, bee pollen may be safe for most individuals. However, ingestion of bee pollen might cause serious reactions in some allergic individuals. Numerous case reports in the medical literature have documented adverse reactions following bee pollen ingestion, including headache, nausea, diarrhea, abdominal pain, and *anaphylaxis,* a life-threatening medical emergency.

Legal and Ethical Aspects

Bee pollen supplementation is legal and ethical.

Recommendations

Bee pollen supplementation is not recommended as a means of improving sports performance. There are no scientific data supporting a sports ergogenic effect. Additionally, bee pollen ingestion might pose a health risk to some individuals. Athletes with allergies should use extreme caution.

Beta-Blockers

Classification and Usage

Beta-blockers may be classified as a pharmacological sports ergogenic. Beta-blockers, also known as *beta-adrenergic blockers,* are prescription drugs designed to depress the stimulant action of epinephrine and norepinephrine on the beta-receptors located in various body tissues, such as the heart. Numerous beta-blockers are available for treating cardiovascular disease and hypertension. A common beta-blocker is propranolol, Inderal being one brand. Beta-blockers are taken about 1–4 hours prior to competition. The dosage depends on the type taken.

Sports Performance Factor

Mental strength. Beta-blockers have been studied in attempts to induce a state of calmness, primarily to decrease the adverse effects of psychological stress during precision sports, such as figure skating, archery, and riflery.

Theory

Excess psychological stress can stimulate the release of epinephrine and norepinephrine, which can increase anxiety, hand tremor, and heart rate. Beta-blockers might enhance precision sports performance by reducing the adverse effects of anxiety on fine motor control, steadying the arm in shooting events through reduction of muscle tremors, and slowing the heart rate so the athlete has more time to fire between heartbeats when the body is not moved slightly by the heart contraction (figure 8.5).

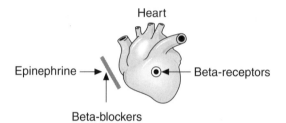

Figure 8.5 Beta-blockers function to inhibit the actions of epinephrine (adrenaline) at various receptors in the body, including the heart.

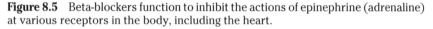

Effectiveness

Research with beta-blockers supports their value as an effective ergogenic aid for the shooting sports. Well-controlled studies with pistol shooters indicate that beta-blockers may decrease anxiety, the feelings of tension, and the emotional increases in heart rate and blood pressure often associated with shooting competition. Pistol shooting performance improved by more than 13 percent, with the improvement attributed to a decrease in muscle tremor and greater steadiness. Research also indicates that beta-blockers may reduce anxiety, as measured by heart rate responses, in high-stress sports such as ski jumping.

Research indicates that beta-blockers may impair several sports performance factors, particularly aerobic endurance capacity in highly trained athletes, probably by depressing the normal stimulant effect of epinephrine. Moreover, use of beta-blockers may impair anaerobic performance in trained athletes, and thus their use is contraindicated.

Safety

Beta-blockers are a useful medication for cardiac and hypertensive patients, but may pose health risks for normal individuals. Adverse side effects include drowsiness, fatigue, nausea, and weakness. Overdoses may cause difficulty in breathing, blood pressure drop, fainting, and possibly congestive heart failure.

Legal and Ethical Aspects

Use of beta-blockers is prohibited for athletes in the 11 pistol and 2 archery events in Olympic competition, as well as in other sports where excess anxiety may interfere with performance, such as bobsledding, luge, freestyle skiing, figure skating, ski jumping, diving, equestrian, fencing, gymnastics, modern pentathlon, sailing, and synchronized swimming. Their use in conjunction with these sports would be unethical.

Recommendations

Although research supports the ergogenic effectiveness of beta-blockers in precision sports such as pistol shooting, they are illegal and may be unsafe; the use of beta-blockers in conjunction with these sports thus cannot be recommended. The use of beta-blockers is not prohibited for other sports, but as noted above, may impair performance in a variety of sports.

Beta-2 Agonists

Classification and Usage

Collectively, *beta-2 agonists* may be classified as pharmacological sports ergogenics. The beta-2 agonist clenbuterol has received considerable media attention as a possible sports ergogenic, but albuterol and other beta-2 agonists have been studied more extensively in humans.

Clenbuterol and other beta-2 agonists are classified as stimulants. *Clenbuterol* is a prescription drug, a beta-2 agonist used for the treatment of asthma in Europe and several other countries. Brand names include Clenasma and Prontovent. The Food and Drug Administration has not approved clenbuterol for use in the United States, although it is attainable through black market sources. *Albuterol* (salbutamol) is an analogous beta-2 agonist approved by the FDA in the United States. Brand names include Proventil and Ventolin.

Clenbuterol is available in aerosol form for inhalation, tablets for oral intake, and solutions for injection. Athletes commonly use the tablet form; the therapeutic dose for asthma treatment is .02 to .03 milligrams twice daily, but athletes have been reported to take twice this amount. Albuterol has been studied primarily in aerosol form. Inhaled doses of 200 to 400 micrograms have been used to evaluate its ergogenic effectiveness.

Sports Performance Factor

Mental strength, physical power, and mechanical edge. Beta-2 agonists have been studied in attempts to enhance various sports performance factors that may benefit from a supplemental mental stimulant effect, including the effects on physical power derived from all three human energy systems, the ATP-CP, lactic acid, and oxygen energy systems.

Additionally, although classified as stimulants, clenbuterol and related beta-2 agonists have been studied in attempts to increase muscle mass for enhanced strength and power or for a more aesthetic physical appearance in sports such as bodybuilding.

Theory

Beta-2 agonists are theorized to enhance pulmonary functions. These drugs stimulate beta-2 receptors in the bronchioli, dilating them and making breathing easier. Theoretically, such an effect would have implications for improving the oxygen energy system, but possible mental stimulant effects of beta-2 agonists could enhance performance of the other energy systems as well.

Although beta-2 agonists are not anabolic/androgenic steroids, some, particularly clenbuterol, are theorized to possess anabolic properties. The underlying mechanism is unknown, but clenbuterol is postulated to affect intracellular enzymes that influence the rate of protein deposition in the muscle. Clenbuterol also may promote lipolysis, or the breakdown of fat in the adipose tissues.

Effectiveness

Several well-controlled studies with inhaled beta-2 agonists, primarily albuterol (salbutamol), have shown evidence of enhanced pulmonary function. These same studies, and others, however, have reported no significant improvement in metabolic or psychological responses to cycle ergometer exercise, a maximal 30-second or 60-second all-out Wingate cycle test of anaerobic capacity, cycle ergometer exercise time to exhaustion, or a simulated 20-kilometer cycle time trial.

Animal studies support the effectiveness of clenbuterol to increase lean muscle mass and reduce fat gain during feeding studies. Individual muscle cell hypertrophy and the increased contractile protein are found in both slow-twitch and fast-twitch muscle fibers.

A recent review reported that there are no experimental human studies with clenbuterol supplementation, particularly humans who are doing resistance training and consuming an adequate diet. Athletes use clenbuterol based on extrapolation of animal research data, but no scientific data support its effectiveness in humans.

Several studies reported that oral beta-2 agonist supplementation, most commonly albuterol, did not increase muscle growth in human subjects involved in resistance strength training, but did increase strength. In one study, 6 measures each of both concentric and eccentric strength performance were evaluated, and albuterol increased performance in 5 of the 12 measures. The mechanism underlying the strength gain has not been determined.

Safety

Nervousness, headaches, muscle tremor, muscle cramps, and heart palpitations are some of the adverse side effects observed in asthma patients using clenbuterol. Similar symptoms have been reported by athletes using clenbuterol illegally. Clenbuterol studies with rats have shown deleterious effects on the heart, a pathological hypertrophy.

Legal and Ethical Aspects

Use of clenbuterol and beta-2 agonists is prohibited by the International Olympic Committee. Interestingly, their use is prohibited as anabolic/androgenic agents, not as stimulants. Clenbuterol use by athletes would be considered unethical.

World champion sprinter Katrin Krabbe received a two-year ban for testing positive for clenbuterol in 1992.

Asthmatic athletes must use legal medications other than oral or injected beta-2 agonists to control asthmatic symptoms because all are prohibited. With medical approval, athletes may use several beta-2 agonists, but in aerosol or inhalant form only because they do not cause systemic effects (protein synthesis, lipolysis) as do the oral or injectable forms. Generic beta-2 agonists salbutamol, salmeterol, and terbutaline may be prescribed by physicians, but athletes should contact their national Olympic committees for guidance.

Recommendations

Although the findings from animal studies are intriguing, no human studies are available to document the effectiveness of clenbuterol as an anabolic agent. Some data indicate beta-2 agonists may increase strength. Health risks of long-term use of anabolic doses in humans have not been determined. Use of clenbuterol and other beta-2 agonists, except those approved for inhalation use, is illegal and unethical. Thus, the use of clenbuterol and other prohibited beta-2 agonists is not recommended. Asthmatic athletes may use approved beta-2 agonist inhalers.

Blood Doping

Classification and Usage

Blood doping, also known as *induced erythrocythemia,* may be classified as a physiological sports ergogenic. Blood doping can be achieved in several ways. One technique is *homologous transfusion,* receipt of blood from another individual whose blood is compatible with the recipient's. In the second method, known as *autologous transfusion,* you receive your own blood, specifically your red blood cells (RBCs), which previously have been withdrawn, frozen, and stored until normal RBC and hemoglobin levels return. In research studies, the amounts of blood or RBCs normally infused have ranged from 500 milliliters to 2 liters, or roughly 1 pint to 2 quarts.

Sports Performance Factor

Physical power. Blood doping has been studied primarily in attempts to increase aerobic power and endurance in sport events that derive energy from the oxygen energy system.

Theory

Blood doping is designed to increase the concentration of RBCs and hemoglobin in the blood. The hemoglobin in the RBC binds with oxygen in the lungs for transport to the muscle; thus, the increased oxygen-carrying capacity of the blood may provide an ergogenic effect for sports involving the oxygen energy system—aerobic power and endurance events of over 5 minutes.

Effectiveness

Several recent major reviews have concluded that blood doping is an effective sports ergogenic for aerobic endurance exercise. Blood or RBC infusions equivalent to 900–2,000 milliliters have been shown to significantly increase total hemoglobin, hemoglobin concentration, RBC mass, and oxygen content in the blood (see figure 8.6). These hematological changes are associated with significant increases in $\dot{V}O_2$max and decreased stress during submaximal exercise, as evidenced by lower heart rates, serum lactates, and psychological ratings of perceived exertion. Exercise performance also is

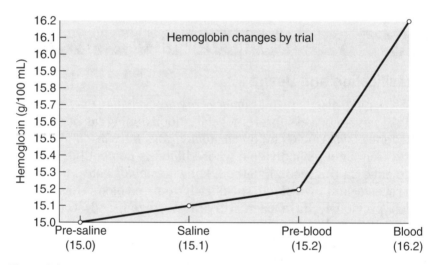

Figure 8.6 Hemoglobin levels increase after blood doping with 2 pints compared to baseline tests and the placebo saline solution.

enhanced by blood doping. Laboratory studies have shown that blood doping increases time to exhaustion in treadmill and cycle ergometer exercise tests and decreases the time to race 5 miles on a treadmill (see figure 8.7); field studies report faster times in races ranging from 1,500 meters to 10,000 meters. Blood doping appears to be one of the most effective sports ergogenics available to athletes.

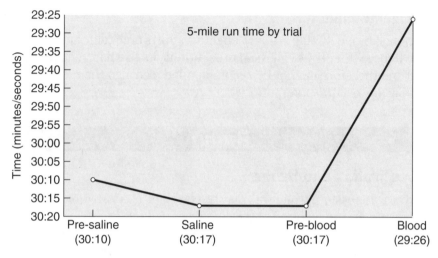

Figure 8.7 Runners improved their 5-mile times by an average of nearly 45 seconds after receiving 2 pints of blood (blood doping).

Safety

Homologous blood transfusions carry risks of hepatitis B, hepatitis C, and HIV (AIDS) infection. Autologous blood transfusions are safer, but clerical error, mislabeling, and mishandling of blood products may cause serious health problems. An incompatible blood transfusion could be fatal.

Legal and Ethical Aspects

Several medal winners on the 1984 United States Olympic cycling team admitted using blood doping procedures prior to the event. Subsequently, blood doping was listed as a prohibited method by the International Olympic Committee in 1985. Current drug testing techniques using urine are unable to detect use of blood doping by an athlete. However, the International Cycling Union recently initiated blood testing and has banned athletes from certain competitions if their hematocrit (percentage of red blood cells) is greater than 50. The use of blood doping as a sports ergogenic is illegal and unethical. The American College of Sports Medicine, an international organization, declared the use of blood doping to improve athletic performance unethical.

Recommendations

Although blood doping is a very effective sports ergogenic and may be safe to use with proper medical precautions, its use has been prohibited and therefore cannot be recommended. See also the recommendations for erythropoietin (EPO).

Boron

Classification and Usage

Boron, a nonessential mineral, may be classified as a nutritional sports ergogenic. Boron is found naturally in many plant foods, particularly dried fruits, nuts, applesauce, and grape juice. No recommended dietary allowance has been developed for boron. However, boron does appear to play some important roles in human metabolism, such as enhancement of bone mineralization, and some scientists suggest it is of nutritional and clinical importance.

Boron supplements are available commercially in tablet form, some targeted to athletes as steroid complexes. Dosages used in human research approximated 2.5 milligrams per day for nearly 2 months.

Sports Performance Factor

Mechanical edge and physical power. Boron supplementation has been studied primarily in attempts to increase muscle mass and decrease body fat for enhanced strength and power or for a more aesthetic physical appearance in sports such as bodybuilding.

Theory

In a study to evaluate the effect of boron supplementation on bone mineralization, postmenopausal women were deprived of boron for 4 months and then provided with a boron supplement for 48 days. One of the effects noted in this study was an increase in serum testosterone levels following the boron supplementation period. Advertisements for boron supplements targeted to athletes soon appeared, suggesting that boron supplementation would increase serum testosterone levels in the body, stimulating anabolic activity with subsequent increases in muscle mass and decreases in body fat.

Effectiveness

Several studies have shown that boron supplementation does not increase serum testosterone levels in either women or men who consume a typical diet. Moreover, research with bodybuilders reported no significant effect of boron supplementation on serum testosterone levels, lean body mass, body fat, or strength. Boron does not appear to be an effective sports ergogenic.

Safety

Although there is no RDA for boron, one scientist suggests that we need to consume about 1 milligram per day, that consumption of 10 milligrams per day is considered safe, and that consumption of 50 milligrams or more per day may be toxic, causing disturbances in appetite and digestion.

Legal and Ethical Aspects

Boron supplements are legal and ethical in conjunction with sport competition.

Recommendations

Based on the available scientific evidence, boron supplementation is not an effective sports ergogenic and hence its use is not recommended.

TABLE 8.4
Foods Rich in Boron (Amounts Containing .5 milligram)

Fruits
Apple sauce (176 grams; 6.2 ounces)
Peaches, canned (267 grams; 9.4 ounces)

Dried fruits
Prunes   (18.5 grams; .65 ounces)
Raisins   (20 grams; .70 ounces)

Vegetables
Broccoli flowers (270 grams; 9.5 ounces)
Parsley flakes   (18.5 grams; .65 ounces)

Nuts
Almonds (21.7 grams; .76 ounces)
Peanuts (27.7 grams; .98 ounces)

Beverages
Wine   (58.8 milliliters; 2 fluid ounces)

However, a leading expert on boron indicated that boron deprivation for 3 weeks or more might have a negative impact on the ability to exercise. Athletes who consume a typical diet should have no problem with boron deprivation. Selecting foods rich in boron, as shown in table 8.4, will help insure adequate boron nutrition.

Branched-Chain Amino Acids (BCAA)

Classification and Usage

Leucine, isoleucine, and valine, the three essential branched-chain amino acids (BCAA), may be classified as nutritional sports ergogenics. The BCAA are natural constituents of protein-rich foods. The Recommended Dietary Allowance for the BCAA is somewhat less than 3 grams per day, which is easily obtainable in the typical diet.

BCAA supplements are commercially available in tablet or powder form, often accompanied by other amino acids. BCAA have been incorporated in sport drinks. Supplementation studies used tablet forms of BCAA ranging from 5 to 20 grams per day, while liquid solutions ranged from about 1 to 7 grams BCAA per liter.

Sports Performance Factor

Mental strength and physical power. BCAA have been studied primarily in attempts to prevent mental fatigue and subsequently enhance performance in very prolonged aerobic endurance exercise tasks, such as distance running, cycling, and even events like prolonged tennis or soccer matches.

Theory

Mental fatigue during exercise is attributed to adverse effects on the central nervous system, primarily the brain, and thus often is referred to as *central fatigue*. Eric Newsholme, a biochemist at Oxford University, proposed that low levels of BCAA in conjunction with high levels of *free-tryptophan (F-tryp)* in the blood could cause central fatigue.

F-tryp is needed for the formation of the brain neurotransmitter serotonin, which may depress the central nervous system and induce symptoms of sleepiness and fatigue. Normally, the amount of F-tryp entering the brain to form serotonin is limited for two reasons. First, high blood levels of BCAA block the entry of F-tryp into the brain (see figure 8.8); and second, tryptophan is normally bound with the blood protein albumin, so it is not free. During the latter stages of prolonged aerobic endurance exercise, F-tryp levels in the blood may gain easier entry to the brain for two reasons. First, as muscle glycogen levels fall, the BCAA levels in the blood might also fall because they may be used to compensate for the decreased energy production from glycogen. Second, free fatty acid levels (FFA), which are bound to albumin for transport in the blood, increase and therefore decrease the amount of albumin available to bind with tryptophan. Thus, a high ratio of F-tryp to BCAA may facilitate the entry of tryptophan into the brain, inducing serotonin formation and causing fatigue. J. Mark Davis has conducted considerable research regarding the central fatigue hypothesis and in a recent review noted there is convincing evidence in support of the

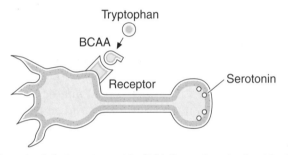

Figure 8.8 Branched chain amino acids (BCAA) are theorized to block the entry of free tryptophan into the brain, decreasing the formation of the neurotransmitter serotonin, which is believed to be partly responsible for fatigue in prolonged aerobic endurance exercise.

theory.

Theoretically, BCAA supplementation would help maintain a more optimal F-tryp to BCAA ratio and prevent the rapid entrance of F-tryp into the brain, thus preventing central fatigue.

Effectiveness

Although the theory underlying the ability of BCAA supplementation to prevent central fatigue is sound, findings of research studies are inconclusive.

On the positive side, when compared to a placebo, acute BCAA supplementation before and during exercise has been shown to increase mental performance following a soccer game and after a 30-kilometer race, and has improved cycling endurance time to exhaustion in the heat. In a study with 193 marathoners, BCAA supplementation did not improve performance overall, but when the runners were subdivided into slower (3:05–3:30 hours:minutes) and faster (<3:05 hours:minutes) groups, the slower runners who received the BCAA ran faster than the slower runners who did not receive the BCAA. The investigators suggested that the slower runners may have depleted their muscle glycogen earlier, thus decreasing blood levels of BCAA earlier in the race and benefiting more from supplementation.

Some research suggests that chronic BCAA supplementation may enhance performance. In a well-designed, double-blind, placebo, cross-over design, researchers at the University of Virginia reported that well-trained cyclists improved their times by 6.8 minutes in a 40-kilometer cycle test following 2 weeks of supplementation, while the improvement following the placebo was only 1.4 minutes.

On the negative side, when compared to a placebo, acute BCAA supplementation before and after exercise has not been shown to improve performance in cycling tests to exhaustion, even when the muscle glycogen levels of the cyclists were depleted. When compared to a glucose supplement in another study, a BCAA-glucose supplementation before and during a 100-kilometer bike performance test decreased the F-tryp:BCAA ratio, but did not improve performance or provide any indication that central fatigue was reduced. Also, in the University of Virginia study cited above, two days of BCAA supplementation had no significant effect on 40-kilometer cycling performance.

Chronic BCAA supplementation, along with other amino acids and nutrients, has not been shown to significantly improve performance in prolonged aerobic endurance exercise at 65 percent $\dot{V}O_2$max or on the total time to complete a half-Ironman type triathlon.

BCAA have been added to carbohydrate solutions in order to study the feasibility of adding BCAA to sport drinks. The usual research protocol involved the use of a placebo, a carbohydrate solution, and a carbohydrate solution with BCAA; one study also used a solution with only BCAA. Several studies have investigated the effects of these solutions on prolonged aerobic exercise tasks of up to 4 hours, and in one study, a 40-kilometer race after hours of cycling. Although both the carbohydrate solution alone and the carbohydrate solution with BCAA improved performance compared to the placebo condition, there were no significant differences between the two. Carbohydrate supplementation may provide adequate energy and diminish the energy contributions of BCAA and FFA, thus preventing a rise in the F-tryp:BCAA ratio and delaying the onset of fatigue.

Safety

BCAA are relatively safe supplements. They include nutrients normally found in protein in the diet. However, some sport nutritionists contend that excess amounts of oral BCAA supplements may inhibit the absorption of other amino acids into the body. Additionally, high doses of BCAA may cause gastrointestinal distress because they may hold water in the intestinal tract. In solution, 7 grams per liter has been used safely.

Legal and Ethical Aspects

BCAA supplements are legal. If they eventually are shown to be effective ergogenics, their use may be considered unethical by some, but currently there does not appear to be an ethical problem with their use in conjunction with sport performance.

Recommendations

Carbohydrate is the primary fuel for prolonged aerobic endurance athletes, and such athletes normally carbohydrate-load before competition and consume carbohydrate beverages during the event. Adding BCAA to the solution does not appear to provide any additional benefits, but neither does it appear to adversely affect prolonged aerobic endurance performance.

Some limited data suggest that chronic BCAA supplementation may benefit performance. One possible theory is that BCAA supplementation may decrease muscle protein breakdown during training, possibly allowing for more consistent training, but carbohydrate supplementation also might be effective in this regard. Adequate dietary protein intake also is essential.

Carbohydrate is the recommended energy source for the aerobic endurance athlete. If carbohydrate nutrition is inadequate, BCAA supplementation may be helpful. Future research may provide better insight into the potential ergogenic effects of BCAA supplementation.

Caffeine

Classification and Usage

Caffeine, a *trimethylxanthine,* may be classified as a pharmacological ergogenic. It also may be considered a nutritional ergogenic because it is a natural constituent of several beverages that are consumed daily, particularly coffee.

A normal therapeutic dose of caffeine is 100–300 milligrams. A 5–6 ounce cup of brewed coffee may contain 100–150 milligrams. Amounts in other products are presented in table 8.5. The purported sports ergogenic effect of some herbal supplements, such as guarana and maté, may be attributed to their caffeine content. The amounts used in research have ranged from 3 to 15 milligrams per kilogram body weight. Thus, a 70-kilogram male might have received amounts ranging from 210 to 1,050 milligrams caffeine.

TABLE 8.5
Typical Caffeine Content in Common Beverages, Pills and Other Products

Brewed coffee, ounce cup* = 100 mg	Excedrin, one tablet = 65 mg
Decaffeinated coffee, cup* = 3 mg	No Doz, one tablet = 100 mg
Medium-brewed tea, cup* = 50 mg	Vivarin, one tablet = 200 mg
Cocoa, cup* = 5 mg	Guarana, 100 milligrams = 100 mg
Cola-type soda, can = 40 mg	
*cup = 5-6 ounces	

Sports Performance Factor

Physical power and mental strength. Caffeine has been studied in attempts to increase physical power from all human energy systems, the ATP-CP, lactic acid, and oxygen energy systems, primarily by its stimulant effects.

Theory

Caffeine is theorized to enhance performance by multiple mechanisms. First, caffeine stimulates the central nervous system and increases psychological arousal, which could enhance performance in a variety of sport events. Second, caffeine stimulates the release of epinephrine from the adrenal gland which, in concert with central nervous system stimulation, may enhance physiological processes such as cardiovascular function and fuel utilization, important during exercise. Regarding fuel utilization, the caffeine-mediated increase in free fatty acid mobilization and the sparing of muscle glycogen is the principal theory underlying the ergogenic effects of caffeine on prolonged aerobic endurance. Third, caffeine facilitates the release of calcium from its storage sites in the muscle cell, enabling calcium to stimulate muscle contraction more effectively. This effect could increase muscular strength and power for short-term, high-intensity exercise tasks dependent primarily on the ATP-CP energy system; power production could be increased in the lactic acid and oxygen energy systems as well. All of these effects may be due to the actions of caffeine, epinephrine, or metabolic byproducts of caffeine breakdown known as dimethylxanthines.

Effectiveness

The sports ergogenic potential of caffeine has been studied for nearly 100 years. Several hundred studies have been conducted, and although the design and the results of individual studies differ, many have shown that caffeine may improve performance in a wide variety of exercise tasks. Table 8.6 highlights some recent research findings supporting an ergogenic effect of caffeine on all three human energy systems.

TABLE 8.6

Improved Performance in the Three Human Energy Systems and in Psychological Arousal Following Caffeine Ingestion

ATP-CP energy system
Maximal power production in 6 seconds
Increased isokinetic strength and power

Lactic acid energy system
100-meter swim

Lactic acid/oxygen energy systems
1,500-meter run

Oxygen system
1,500-meter swim
Cycle and run time to exhaustion > 60 minutes

Psychological arousal
Increased work output at a set rating of perceived exertion

Several recent reviews by internationally known investigators such as Lawrence Spriet and Terry Graham, of contemporary well-controlled studies, conclude that caffeine may be an effective sports ergogenic even when consumed in legal amounts. (See the legal and ethical aspects.) This is particularly so for aerobic power and endurance events dependent on the oxygen energy system, but caffeine also may benefit events somewhat dependent on power endurance. Thus, if we use track events as an example, caffeine may improve performance in events such as 1,500 meters, 5,000 meters, and the marathon (42.2 kilometers). Extrapolation of other exercise performance data suggests caffeine also may be an effective ergogenic for shorter track events, such as 100 and 400 meters, but these data are less convincing than those for longer distances.

Although these reviewers indicate caffeine may enhance physical performance, most studies have been conducted in the laboratory or under noncompetitive situations. Thus, it may be possible that the stress of actual sport competition influences epinephrine levels to the extent that any additive effect of caffeine is nullified. For example, one study revealed that 5 to 9 milligrams of caffeine per kilogram body weight did not improve performance of endurance-trained runners in a 13.1-mile (21.1-kilometer) half-marathon under heat-stress conditions. More research is needed to evaluate the effectiveness of caffeine as a sports ergogenic when used in actual or simulated sport competition.

Safety

Caffeine is relatively safe for healthy athletes. Over-consumption may cause caffeinism with possible side effects of flushing of the face, nervousness, trembling, anxiety, and heart palpitations. People with various health problems, such as high blood pressure, should consult their physicians regarding caffeine use.

Legal and Ethical Aspects

Caffeine is classified as a stimulant by the International Olympic Committee. Although the use of most stimulants is prohibited, some caffeine is allowed because it is a natural constituent of beverages consumed by athletes. Excess amounts of caffeine leading to urine levels of 12 micrograms caffeine/milliliter urine or above are grounds for disqualification. The USOC notes that intake of 100 milligrams of caffeine will result in a urine profile of 1.5 micrograms/milliliter. Thus, 800 milligrams would be needed to reach the illegal level. The amount needed to reach the illegal level may vary depending on body weight, gender, and body water levels. For some athletes, a dose much lower than 800 milligrams of caffeine could exceed the legal limit. The following amounts of caffeine-containing products could exceed the legal limit:

8 cups of perked coffee

16–20 cans of cola-type soda

8 NoDoz tablets

4 Vivarin tablets

12 Excedrin tablets

The ergogenic effects of caffeine are present . . . at levels . . . allowed by the IOC. This raises serious ethical issues regarding the use of caffeine to improve athletic performance.

—*Lawrence Spriet, Canadian exercise physiologist*

Recommendations

Caffeine appears to be an effective sports ergogenic, even when consumed in doses that are considered legal. Caffeine also is relatively safe. However, some investigators have suggested caffeine use may be unethical and have recommended that the IOC consider lowering the urinary level considered to be illegal. Currently, the decision whether to use caffeine is up to the individual athlete.

If you decide to use caffeine, a recommended dose may be 5 milligrams per kilogram body weight. One kilogram equals 2.2 pounds, so a 60-kilogram (132-pound) distance runner would consume 300 milligrams. Some preliminary research shows that caffeine pills, such as Vivarin, may be more effective than caffeine found in coffee; thus, one to two Vivarin tablets would provide 200 to 400 milligrams caffeine. If you prefer coffee, 2 to 3 cups should be sufficient. Five milligrams per kilogram body weight has been found to be just as effective as higher doses, but has not been shown to elevate urine levels to 12 micrograms/milliliter. Abstaining from caffeine-containing beverages for 2 to 3 days prior to competition also might help. Some, but not all, studies indicate abstention may enhance the effect of caffeine to stimulate epinephrine release.

Individuals may respond differently to caffeine and those susceptible to some of its side effects, such as nervousness and trembling, may experience an impairment in sports performance.

Calcium

Classification and Usage

Calcium, an essential mineral, may be classified as a nutritional sports ergogenic. Calcium is a natural constituent of various foods, particularly dairy products, dark-green leafy vegetables, and legumes. Some foods, such as orange juice, are fortified with calcium. The Recommended Dietary Allowance is 800 milligrams for adults and 1,200 milligrams for those aged 11 to 25.

Calcium supplements are available in a variety of forms, including calcium carbonate and calcium gluconate. Tums, an antacid, also contains calcium. Supplements of 200 milligrams are normally taken with meals.

Sports Performance Factor

Physical power. Calcium supplementation may be used primarily in attempts to increase physical power from all three human energy systems, the ATP-CP, lactic acid, and oxygen energy systems.

Theory

Almost all (99 percent) of the calcium in the body is stored in the bones and teeth, but the remaining 1 percent in other tissues is essential for numerous metabolic functions. In particular, calcium is essential for contraction of all muscles in the body, so a deficiency could impair performance in almost any type of sport activity. Calcium also activates a number of enzymes important to sport performance, including enzymes that break down muscle glycogen for energy production.

Effectiveness

There are no scientific data supporting an ergogenic effect of calcium supplementation. The body possesses a powerful hormonal system to help maintain normal calcium levels in the tissues. Thus, when tissue levels begin to get low, hormones mobilize excess calcium from the bones for delivery to the tissues. The amounts taken from the bones may be restored later through dietary sources.

Safety

Calcium supplementation to help achieve a total dietary intake of 800 to 1,200 milligrams appears to be safe. Excessive calcium intake may cause constipation or interfere with the absorption of other essential minerals, such as iron and zinc. In some susceptible individuals, excess calcium intake may contribute to the development of kidney stones or irregular heartbeats.

Legal and Ethical Aspects

Calcium supplements are legal and ethical.

Recommendations

In general, calcium supplementation is not recommended as a sports ergogenic because it has not been found to effectively enhance sport performance.

Athletes ideally should obtain adequate calcium through their diet, selecting foods rich in calcium as noted in table 8.7. If foods are not

---

TABLE 8.7
Calcium Content of Common Foods in the Various Food Groups and Fast Foods

Milk
1 cup 1 percent fat milk = 300 milligrams
1 cup nonfat yogurt = 350 milligrams

Meat/fish/poultry/cheese
1 ounce Swiss cheese = 270 milligrams
1 ounce lean steak = 3 milligrams
1 ounce shrimp = 11 milligrams

Breads/cereals/legumes/starchy vegetables
1 slice whole-wheat bread = 18 milligrams
1 cup baked beans = 127 milligrams
1 cup corn = 8 milligrams

Vegetables
1 cup cooked broccoli = 70 milligrams
1 cup cooked spinach = 245 milligrams

Fruits
1 banana = 6 milligrams
1/4 cup raisins = 18 milligrams

Fast foods
1 Burger King BK broiler = 60 milligrams
1 Pizza Hut medium slice pan cheese pizza = 250 milligrams

selected wisely, some athletes might benefit from calcium supplements, including (a) those who abstain from dairy products, (b) those who participate in weight-control sports, (c) young females who become amenorrheic, and (d) older females. In such cases, the recommended procedure is to supplement the normal calcium intake with about 200 milligrams, three times per day with meals, to obtain total intakes ranging from 800 to 1,500 milligrams.

Calcium supplementation is not ergogenic per se, but may help in the prevention of premature osteoporosis, particularly in young athletes but also in older athletes. Osteoporosis weakens the bones and makes them more susceptible to stress fractures or even complete fractures.

Carbohydrate Supplements

Classification and Usage

Carbohydrate supplements may be classified as a nutritional sports ergogenic. Dietary carbohydrates are found naturally in many foods we eat and come in a variety of forms, often collectively known as *simple carbohydrates* (sugars) and *complex carbohydrates* (starches). Glucose and fructose, two of the most basic simple sugars, are found naturally in many fruits. Sucrose (common table sugar) and lactose (milk sugar) also are simple carbohydrates. Starches, found in grains and vegetables, are complex carbohydrates formed from long chains of glucose. Sucrose is a manufactured sugar, as are high-fructose corn syrup and glucose polymers, the latter being a chain of more than 10 glucose molecules. No Recommended Dietary Allowance has been established for carbohydrate, but dieticians indicate it should constitute about 55 percent to 60 percent of the daily caloric intake, or even higher in many athletes.

The major function of carbohydrate in the human body is to provide energy. The role of carbohydrate as an energy source for both the lactic acid and oxygen energy systems was discussed previously.

Numerous commercial carbohydrate supplements marketed to athletes include sport drinks, sport bars, glucose tablets, concentrated sugar gels, and glucose polymer powders. The types and amounts of carbohydrates used in research have varied in attempts to determine those most useful for improving sports performance.

Many recommendations for carbohydrate supplementation are given in grams. Most food labels will list the grams of carbohydrate per serving, so this is an easy way to determine daily intake in grams, although you will need to subtract the dietary fiber sources. When it is recommended that you consume 60 percent of your daily calories from carbohydrate, simply take 60 percent of your daily caloric intake and divide by 4; this will provide you with an estimate of the grams of carbohydrate you should consume daily. For example, an athlete who consumes 3,000 calories per day would need 450 grams of carbohydrate. To do the math, multiply .60 times 3,000 calories, which equals 1,800 calories from carbohydrate. Each gram of carbohydrate equals 4 calories, so divide the 1,800 calories by 4, which equals 450 grams.

Sports Performance Factor

Physical power. Carbohydrate supplementation is used in attempts to increase aerobic power and endurance for sport events that derive energy primarily from the oxygen energy system, but may also be useful in prolonged, intermittent, high-intensity anaerobic sports such as soccer.

Theory

Carbohydrate is the primary energy source when exercising above 65 percent of VO_2max during prolonged aerobic exercise. It is a more efficient fuel compared to fat; that is, you produce more ATP per unit of oxygen consumed when oxidizing carbohydrate compared to fat. The body contains only limited amounts of carbohydrate stored as muscle glycogen, liver glycogen, and blood glucose. When carbohydrate levels become insufficient, fatigue may occur because: (a) depleted muscle glycogen levels increase the reliance on fat as an energy source which decreases ATP production, thus slowing the pace; (b) depleted liver glycogen stores reduce the amount of blood glucose, thus depriving the muscle of a source of carbohydrate energy; (c) decreased blood glucose levels (hypoglycemia) may deprive the brain of its primary energy source, thus impairing normal brain function and causing weakness and disorientation; or (d) inadequate muscle glycogen and blood glucose may interfere with amino acid metabolism in the brain, causing fatigue by production of serotonin, a depressant neurotransmitter. (See central nervous system fatigue theory, discussed under BCAA.)

Carbohydrate, as muscle glycogen, is the only source of energy in the lactic acid energy system that is used predominantly during high-intensity, anaerobic exercise.

Carbohydrate supplementation theoretically would enhance prolonged aerobic endurance exercise performance by providing optimal carbohydrate storage as muscle glycogen and liver glycogen and by helping to maintain optimal blood glucose levels. Carbohydrate supplementation also might enhance performance in prolonged, intermittent, high-intensity anaerobic sports by increased storage of muscle glycogen in or delivery of glucose to the fast-twitch (FT) muscle fibers.

Effectiveness

Carbohydrate supplementation and its effect on sport performance is the most studied sports ergogenic. Thousands of studies and scores of reviews have evaluated its effectiveness for improving performance in a variety of sport endeavors. Almost all reviewers indicate that carbohydrate supplementation is a very effective sports ergogenic for helping to delay the onset of fatigue, but only if the carbohydrate supplement prevents the premature depletion of normal body carbohydrate stores, depletion of which would induce fatigue.

In general, research supports the following conclusions relative to the effectiveness of carbohydrate supplementation as a sports ergogenic.

1. Carbohydrate supplementation will not enhance performance in aerobic endurance events lasting less than 60 minutes, provided the athlete has normal levels of muscle and liver glycogen at the beginning.

2. Carbohydrate supplementation may improve performance in more prolonged aerobic endurance events, particularly those 90 minutes or more. Marathon running (42.2 kilometers, 26.2 miles), century cycle trials (162 kilometers, 100 miles), and long-distance triathlons are examples. Although athletes might not go faster during the early stages of these events, carbohydrate supplementation enables them to maintain an optimal pace for a longer time, thus completing the race in less time.

3. Carbohydrate supplementation may improve performance in prolonged, intermittent, high-intensity sport endeavors such as soccer, field hockey, and tennis. Research has shown that carbohydrate supplementation may enable soccer players to run more and faster during the latter stages of the second half and to score more and concede fewer goals.

Safety

Carbohydrate supplements are considered safe. Excess consumption of some simple carbohydrates, particularly fructose, or glucose polymers, may create an osmotic effect and draw excess water into the intestine, causing diarrhea.

Legal and Ethical Aspects

Carbohydrate supplementation is legal and ethical in conjunction with sport competition.

Recommendations

Many athletes do not consume enough carbohydrate on a day-to-day basis. Thus, a basic recommendation for all athletes, particularly endurance athletes, is a diet that stresses wholesome foods rich in natural simple and complex carbohydrates; in addition to carbohydrate, you get vitamins, minerals, some protein, and other substances with potential health benefits, such as fiber. Natural foods rich in carbohydrates are found primarily in the starch/bread, fruit, and vegetable food exchanges.

Approximately 60 percent to 70 percent of daily dietary calories should be derived from carbohydrates within the various food exchanges. For athletes who consume high-calorie diets daily, a somewhat lower percentage may provide adequate dietary carbohydrates. An athlete who consumes 4,000 calories per day with 50 percent derived from carbohydrate would obtain 500 grams of carbohydrate, a rather substantial amount. Athletes on weight-loss diets should stay at 60 percent of the calories from carbohydrate, or somewhat lower, to ensure adequate protein and fat in the diet.

Table 8.8 presents the carbohydrate content in grams per serving of some basic food exchanges, along with the number of calories per serving; the additional calories are derived from the carbohydrate and/or fat content in the food. A balanced diet containing many of these high-carbohydrate foods will help to ensure adequate body reserves of liver and muscle glycogen for sustained high-intensity anaerobic and aerobic training.

Although wholesome, natural foods are the best way to obtain dietary carbohydrate, use of commercial carbohydrate supplements may be convenient under certain circumstances, such as for snacks and during sports competition. It is important to emphasize that carbohydrate supplements should be used as an adjunct to an otherwise balanced nutritional plan, not as a substitute.

In general, research supports the following recommendations relative to carbohydrate intake in conjunction with training and competition for sports in which depleted body carbohydrate sources may

---

TABLE 8.8

Grams of Carbohydrate and Calories Per Serving for the
Basic Food Exchanges

Skim/very-low-fat milk—12 grams carbohydrate and 90 calories per serving

1 cup skim milk	1 cup plain, low-fat yogurt

Starchy vegetables, legumes, breads, cereals—15 grams carbohydrate and 80 calories per serving

1/2 cup cooked or dry cereal	1 small baked potato
1/2 cup cooked pasta	1/3 cup baked beans
1/2 cup cooked grits	1/2 cup corn
1/3 cup cooked rice	1/2 English muffin
1/2 bagel	3/4 ounce pretzels
1 slice bread	6 saltine crackers

Vegetables—5 grams carbohydrate and 25 calories per serving

1/2 cup cooked vegetables	1/2 cup vegetable juice
1 cup raw vegetables	

Examples: carrots, green beans, broccoli, cauliflower, onions, spinach, tomatoes, tomato juice

Fruits—15 grams carbohydrate and 60 calories per serving

1 small apple	1/2 banana

Other carbohydrates—15 grams carbohydrate and 60 calories per serving

2 small fat-free cookies	3 gingersnaps
1 tablespoon fruit spread	1/2 cup frozen fat-free yogurt

Note: Adapted from Exchange Lists for Meal Planning by the American Diabetes Association and American Dietetic Association, 1995, Alexandria, VA: American Diabetes Association and Chicago: American Dietetic Association

---

predispose athletes to premature fatigue. Because every individual may react differently, however, it is important that you experiment with various carbohydrate types and amounts in training before use in actual competition in order to avoid any adverse reactions.

Carbohydrate Intake Before Exercise

1. To be used as an energy source during exercise, ingested carbohydrate needs to empty from the stomach into the intestines and be

absorbed into the bloodstream for transport to the muscles. In this regard, studies have investigated the ergogenic effects of various types (glucose, fructose, sucrose, glucose polymers), forms (solid, gels, liquid), and glycemic index (high, low).

In general, there are no differences among the various forms, types, or glycemic indices as a means of supplying carbohydrates to enhance physical performance. Some recent research suggests low-glycemic index foods may supply carbohydrates for a longer time during exercise, but more research is needed to support any additional ergogenic effect above that provided by high-glycemic index foods.

2. The amount of carbohydrate you consume before exercise is dependent on your body weight; the following are prudent recommendations.

a. 4 hours before exercise: 4 grams per kilogram body weight

b. 1 hour before exercise: 1 gram per kilogram body weight

c. 10 minutes before exercise: .5 gram per kilogram body weight

For example, if you weigh 65 kilograms (143 pounds), you would consume 260 grams of carbohydrate 4 hours before exercise, 65 grams 1 hour before exercise, or about 35 grams just before exercise.

Carbohydrate Intake During Exercise

1. Although your muscles may be able to oxidize 200 grams of carbohydrate or more per hour, research suggests that athletes may be able to use only about 30 to 60 grams of carbohydrate ingested during each hour of exercise. Eight fluid ounces (about 240 milliliters) of a typical sport drink (about 6 percent carbohydrate) provides almost 15 grams of carbohydrate. Thus, drinking this amount every 15 minutes will provide you with 60 grams per hour (figure 8.9).

You may wish to experiment with sport drinks containing higher concentrations of carbohydrate if you desire less fluid. The amount of carbohydrate in commercial sport drinks varies. Gatorade is a 5–6 percent solution, while others may be as high as 10 percent. If you want to try preparing your own sport drink, dry glucose polymers are available in many sporting goods stores. To make a solution of a given percentage, you need to put a certain amount (dry ounces) of the polymer powder into a certain amount (fluid ounces) of water. You can use a measuring cup to measure ounces. Two ounces of dry powder in a quart of water (32 ounces) will produce a solution of about 6 percent

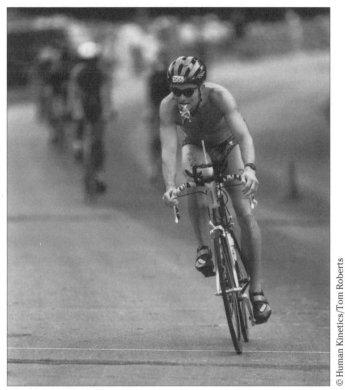

Figure 8.9 Carbohydrate intake during prolonged aerobic endurance exercise has been shown to be an effective way to enhance performance.

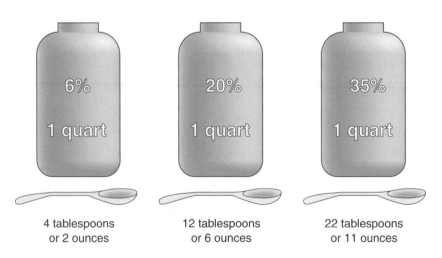

6% 1 quart	20% 1 quart	35% 1 quart
4 tablespoons or 2 ounces	12 tablespoons or 6 ounces	22 tablespoons or 11 ounces

Figure 8.10 How to make a 6 percent, 20 percent, or 35 percent glucose-polymer solution.

(2/32 =.0625). If you put 1 level tablespoon (.5 ounce) of the polymer in a glass of water (8 ounces), you will have about a 6 percent to 7 percent solution (.5/8 =.0625). Figure 8.10 illustrates how to make a 6 percent, a 20 percent, and a 35 percent solution using a quart of water for each. You also can follow the directions usually found on the commercial products.

2. When exercising under warm or hot environmental conditions, carbohydrates in fluids is the recommended approach to providing carbohydrate for energy and fluids for temperature regulations. See Fluid Supplementation (Sport Drinks) and table 8.9 to calculate carbohydrate and fluid needs during exercise.

TABLE 8.9
Milliliters of Fluid Supplementation at 6%, 8%, and 10% Concentration to Provide 30 to 60 Grams of Carbohydrate

Percent concentration	GRAMS OF CARBOHYDRATE			
	30	40	50	60
6%	500	666	833	1,000
8%	375	500	625	750
10%	300	400	500	600

Carbohydrate Intake After Exercise

1. For athletes who train intensely on a daily basis, including high-intensity resistance, anaerobic, or aerobic exercise, carbohydrate intake following exercise is needed to help return body carbohydrate stores to normal. Consuming a high-carbohydrate diet, about 60 percent to 70 percent or more of the daily calories as carbohydrate, should help restore muscle and liver glycogen to normal levels and help you maintain high-intensity workouts as needed on the following day.

One recommendation is to obtain 8 to 10 grams of carbohydrate per kilogram body weight over a 24-hour period. For a 65-kilogram athlete, this would represent 520 to 650 grams of carbohydrate, or about 2,080 to 2,600 carbohydrate calories per day. On a 3,500-calorie diet this represents about 60 percent to 75 percent of the daily calories from carbohydrate.

About 500 grams of carbohydrate in the daily diet

6 slices of whole wheat bread (90 grams)

2 cups of cooked pasta (60 grams)

2 glasses of skim milk (24 grams)

2 bananas (60 grams)

1 baked potato, medium (30 grams)

1 apple (15 grams)

6 gingersnaps (30 grams)

2 small bagels (60 grams)

1 cup dry cereal (30 grams)

1/2 cup baked beans (15 grams)

1 cup orange juice (30 grams)

1 cup pineapple juice (30 grams)

1/4 cup canned peaches (15 grams)

1 ounce pretzels (20 grams)

2. To speed up glycogen synthesis following exercise, athletes should consume about 1 gram of carbohydrate per kilogram body weight within 15 minutes afterward and repeat this procedure every 2 hours for the next 4 to 6 hours. In this case, our 65-kilogram athlete would consume 65 grams of carbohydrate four times within six hours after exercising. The high carbohydrate meals increase and maintain insulin levels to help promote muscle and liver glycogen synthesis.

3. Some research suggests that combining protein with carbohydrates following exercise will speed up muscle glycogen synthesis even more than carbohydrate alone. Insulin is also an anabolic hormone and may help inhibit protein catabolism after resistance exercise.

The ratio of carbohydrate to protein, in grams, should be about 3 to 1. If we use the values above, a 65-kilogram athlete would consume 65 grams of carbohydrate and about 21 grams of protein, about a 3:1 ratio. These amounts could be derived easily through natural foods, such as milk, bananas, and cereal. Some sport drinks also contain protein in addition to carbohydrate, and could be a convenient way of using this technique. For example, one can of GatorPro contains nearly 60 grams of carbohydrate and 17 grams of protein.

Carbohydrate-Loading

A full program of carbohydrate-loading may be recommended for major competitions, such as a 42.2-kilometer marathon, a 100-mile bike ride, or a 2- or 3-day soccer tournament. Table 8.10 presents a recommended format for a 1-week carbohydrate-loading regimen. On day 1, you should engage in a prolonged, but not exhaustive, exercise bout to reduce the amount of glycogen in the liver and muscles. This exercise task is followed by 3 days of tapering exercise and moderate carbohydrate intake and then 3 days of tapering exercise or rest and high carbohydrate intake (approximately 8 to 10 grams of carbohydrate per kilogram body weight per day, or 500 to 600 grams).

Table 8.8 presents some guidelines to the gram carbohydrate content of various high-carbohydrate foods. These foods should be stressed in the daily diet along with about 6-8 ounces of lean meat, poultry, or fish to guarantee high-quality protein. The food listed in the sidebar, if consumed in the main meals and snacks throughout the day, will provide more than 500 grams of carbohydrate.

TABLE 8.10
Recommended Carbohydrate-Loading Regimen

Day 1 Moderately long exercise bout (should not be exhaustive)
Day 2 Mixed diet; moderate carbohydrate intake; tapering exercise
Day 3 Mixed diet; moderate carbohydrate intake; tapering exercise
Day 4 Mixed diet; moderate carbohydrate intake; tapering exercise
Day 5 High carbohydrate diet; tapering exercise
Day 6 High carbohydrate diet; tapering exercise or rest
Day 7 High carbohydrate diet; tapering exercise or rest
Day 8 Competition

Note: The moderate carbohydrate diet intake should approximate 200 to 300 grams of carbohydrate per day; the high carbohydrate intake should approximate 500 to 600 grams of carbohydrate per day. Actual carbohydrate intake may depend on body weight. See text for more information.

Carnitine (L-Carnitine)

Classification and Usage

Carnitine is a dietary supplement that may be classified as a physiological sports ergogenic. The biologically active form in the body is L-Carnitine. Although L-Carnitine is a vitamin-like substance, it is not considered an essential nutrient because it may be formed in the body from several amino acids. Primary dietary sources of carnitine include meat and milk products. Commercial L-Carnitine products are sold separately or in combination with other purported nutritional sports ergogenics. Dosages used in research have ranged from .5 to 6 grams per day taken for periods ranging from 1 day to 4 weeks.

Sports Performance Factor

Physical power. L-Carnitine has been studied primarily in attempts to increase power endurance and aerobic power and endurance in events associated with both the lactic acid and oxygen energy systems.

Theory

L-Carnitine, as a cofactor for several enzymes in the muscle cell, may influence the metabolism of fatty acids and energy substrate for the Krebs cycle in several ways that may have important implications for sports performance.

L-Carnitine supplementation may influence fatty acid metabolism, facilitating the transfer of long-chain fatty acids into the mitochondria for energy production. Increased oxidation of fatty acids could decrease the use of carbohydrates as an energy source, sparing muscle glycogen for the latter stages of prolonged aerobic endurance events.

Additionally, other metabolic effects of L-Carnitine could facilitate the entrance of pyruvate (a byproduct of glucose breakdown) into the mitochondria for energy production. Theoretically, L-Carnitine supplementation could decrease the accumulation of lactic acid and improve anaerobic power endurance.

Conversely, some investigators theorize that L-Carnitine supplementation might impair prolonged aerobic endurance performance by increasing glucose metabolism; an increased utilization of pyruvate could lead to a premature depletion of muscle glycogen.

Effectiveness

For L-Carnitine supplementation to be effective, muscle carnitine levels must increase. L-Carnitine supplementation will increase plasma levels of L-Carnitine in humans, but muscle L-Carnitine levels do not appear to be affected following supplementation with 4 to 6 grams for 2 weeks. One study, however, reported increased muscle L-Carnitine levels following 6 months supplementation with 2 grams per day.

L-Carnitine supplementation does not appear to reduce lactic acid accumulation during strenuous exercise. This finding has been documented by numerous well-controlled studies measuring blood lactate levels following such exercise tasks as a 600-meter run, a 4-minute high-velocity run, a 5-kilometer run, and repeated 1-minute high-intensity cycle performance tests.

The effect of L-Carnitine supplementation on oxidation of fatty acids during exercise is unresolved. Two studies have found a reduced respiratory exchange ratio (RER), a marker for increased fatty acid oxidation during submaximal exercise following L-Carnitine supplementation. Several other studies, however, using strategies such as a fat-loading diet or depletion of muscle glycogen to facilitate use of fatty acids as an energy source, did not report any effect of L-Carnitine on the RER.

The effect of L-Carnitine supplementation on $\dot{V}O_2$max is also equivocal. Two studies have shown improvements in $\dot{V}O_2$max up to 6 percent following supplementation with 4 grams per day for 2 weeks; three other studies reported no significant effect with 2 to 3 grams per day for 1 to 4 weeks.

When used to correct an L-Carnitine deficiency in humans, physical performance is often improved. There are no studies indicating L-Carnitine supplementation enhances physical power in healthy individuals for events associated with either the lactic acid or oxygen energy systems. Well-controlled studies found that L-Carnitine supplementation did not improve power endurance in repeat 91.4-meter (100-yard) swims in male collegiate swimmers (lactic acid energy system), or aerobic power in a 5-kilometer treadmill run time in competitive male distance runners (oxygen energy system).

There are no studies evaluating the effect of L-Carnitine supplementation on prolonged aerobic endurance exercise tasks that may benefit from muscle glycogen sparing. Muscle glycogen sparing is one of the main theories underlying L-Carnitine supplementation, and this theory needs to be researched to evaluate its validity.

Safety

Pharmacological grade L-Carnitine supplementation appears to be safe. Studies using doses of 2 to 6 grams daily for up to a month have not shown any adverse side effects. Larger doses may cause diarrhea. One investigator noted there are few data regarding health risks of chronic supplementation with high dosages. Additionally, the purity of commercial L-Carnitine supplements may vary. D,L-Carnitine should not be used because it might interfere with normal L-Carnitine functions in the body.

Legal and Ethical Aspects

Carnitine supplementation is legal and ethical.

Recommendations

Carnitine supplementation is not recommended as a way to improve sports performance. There are inadequate scientific data on actual physical performance to support a sports ergogenic effect. Some, but not all, data indicate L-Carnitine supplementation may enhance fatty acid oxidation, which could benefit performance in very prolonged aerobic endurance exercise tasks. Endurance athletes prone to low levels of muscle L-Carnitine (vegetarians who consume no animal products) might benefit from L-Carnitine supplementation.

Choline (Lecithin)

Classification and Usage

Choline is a dietary supplement that may be classified as a physiological sports ergogenic; some might classify it as a nutritional sports ergogenic. Although choline is a vitamin-like substance, it is not considered an essential nutrient because its metabolic role in the body can be assumed by other dietary nutrients. Primary dietary sources of choline include lecithin (phosphatidylcholine) in animal foods such as egg yolks and organ meats such as liver, and free choline in plants, especially nuts, wheat germ, cauliflower, spinach, and soybeans. Dietary intake is approximately .4 to .9 gram per day, enough to meet the body's needs.

Commercial choline products are available as lecithin or choline salts. The actual choline in commercial products varies because choline is only one part of lecithin compounds and choline salts.

Check labels for actual choline content. Choline also is marketed as a powder with carbohydrate and electrolytes, such as Pro Enhancer, which is designed to be concocted as a sport drink. Dosages used in research have ranged from about 2.5 to 5.0 grams of choline salts and up to 14 grams of lecithin, usually consumed about an hour before exercise.

Sports Performance Factor

Physical power. Choline has been studied primarily in attempts to increase aerobic endurance in events associated with the oxygen energy system.

Theory

Choline is important to human metabolism in a variety of ways, but has been theorized to be a sports ergogenic because of its involvement in the formation of acetylcholine, an important neurotransmitter in the central nervous system and at the junction between the nerve and the muscle. Acetylcholine release starts the muscle contraction process. Several studies have shown that blood choline levels decrease following prolonged aerobic endurance exercise, such as marathon running. Choline supplementation theoretically would help maintain normal acetylcholine levels for optimal neural and muscular function.

Effectiveness

Research has shown rather conclusively that choline salt or lecithin supplementation will increase blood choline levels at rest and during prolonged exercise. This effect may be ergogenic. For example, some preliminary field and laboratory research suggested choline supplementation significantly decreased the time to run 20 miles and improved mood states of cyclists 40 minutes after completion of a cycle ergometer ride to exhaustion. On the other hand, well-controlled laboratory research has revealed that choline supplementation exerted no effect on either brief, high-intensity anaerobic cycling tests lasting about 2 minutes, or on more prolonged aerobic exercise tasks lasting about 70 minutes.

These findings are equivocal and substantiate the need for more research with choline supplementation, particularly controlled laboratory research involving prolonged aerobic endurance exercise tasks greater than 2 hours in duration.

In other research, choline supplementation has not been found to increase performance in rifle-shooting accuracy in biathlon-type events, indicating choline supplementation has no anxiolytic effect.

Safety

No adverse side effects were noted in the studies employing choline salt or lecithin supplementation totaling approximately 1.5 to 2.0 grams of choline.

Legal and Ethical Aspects

Choline supplementation is legal and ethical. If choline salts or lecithin eventually are shown to be effective ergogenics, some might consider their use to be unethical.

Recommendations

Choline supplementation is legal, safe, and ethical. However, the scientific data regarding its effectiveness as a sports ergogenic are equivocal. Thus, choline supplementation cannot be recommended.

Nevertheless, some investigators noted high-carbohydrate diets consumed by many endurance athletes might not contain large quantities of foods rich in choline and endurance athletes might deplete body stores through daily, prolonged endurance exercise. The ideal solution is to consume more dietary choline (egg yolks, organ meats, spinach, cauliflower, nuts, and wheat germ), but choline supplements might be helpful. More well-controlled research is needed to resolve this issue.

Chromium

Classification and Usage

Chromium, an essential mineral, may be classified as a nutritional sports ergogenic. Chromium is found naturally in foods, particularly whole-grain products, cheese, nuts, brewer's yeast, and vegetables such as mushrooms and asparagus. The estimated safe and adequate daily dietary intake (ESADDI) of chromium is 50 to 200 micrograms.

Chromium supplements are available in various salt forms, including chromium picolinate and chromium nicotinate. Dosages used in human research approximated 200 to 400 micrograms per day for several months.

In a recent survey of magazines targeted to body-builders, chromium was one of the top two dietary supplements advertised.

Sports Performance Factor

Mechanical edge and physical power. Chromium supplementation has been studied primarily in attempts to increase muscle mass and decrease body fat for enhanced strength and power or for a more aesthetic physical appearance in sports such as bodybuilding. Chromium also may be used in attempts to improve performance in prolonged aerobic endurance exercise tasks.

Theory

Chromium is part of a biologically active organic complex in the body known as the *glucose tolerance factor (GTF)* that is believed to enhance insulin sensitivity. Theoretically, chromium supplementation will enhance the anabolic activity of insulin, increasing muscle mass by promoting the transfer of amino acids into the muscle cell, stimulating protein synthesis, and decreasing the rate of muscle protein breakdown (figure 8.11). An enhanced insulin sensitivity might influence the hunger center in the hypothalamus, reducing food intake and eventually decreasing body fat. Advertisements claim chromium supplements may be an alternative to the use of anabolic/androgenic steroids.

Increased insulin sensitivity may enhance the storage of muscle and liver glycogen and may improve utilization of glucose during exercise, factors that theoretically could enhance performance in prolonged aerobic endurance events.

Effectiveness

Animal research indicates that chronic chromium supplementation to young animals during their growth periods increases lean muscle tissue and decreases body fat. Research findings regarding the effects of short-term chromium supplementation on the body composition of adult humans are less abundant and less clear. Early research findings with college students and football players suggested that chromium supplementation over a 12-week period could increase lean muscle mass. These studies have been criticized for improper methodology

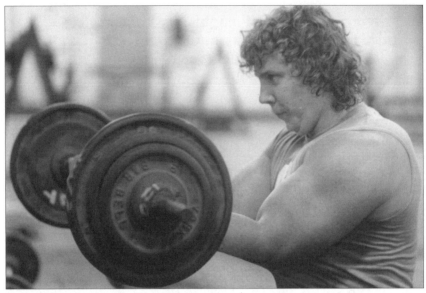

Figure 8.11 Chromium supplements are popular among bodybuilders for their purported value in decreasing body fat and increasing muscle mass. However, research is not very supportive.

because they used less reliable means to determine body composition and did not control or assess dietary intake of the subjects.

In more contemporary research, several investigators replicated those earlier studies. Using more valid techniques to assess body composition and evaluate the dietary intake of the subjects, they reported no significant effect of chromium supplementation on lean body mass, body fat, or muscular strength and endurance.

Although chromium supplementation may be theorized to enhance prolonged aerobic endurance capacity by favorably affecting glucose metabolism, no research has studied this issue.

The more well-designed studies do not support the effectiveness of chromium supplementation as a means to improve body composition or muscular function for sport competition, and no data support an ergogenic effect on prolonged aerobic endurance exercise.

Safety

Chromium supplementation in amounts no larger than the estimated safe and adequate daily dietary intake (ESADDI) of 50 to 200 micrograms appears to be safe. Larger doses have been used in the treatment of diabetes. A recent research review suggested that chronic supplementation with certain forms of chromium supplements, such as chromium picolinate, may lead to chromium accumulation in the body to the levels at which DNA damage has been observed in animals. Some scientists recommend that the chronic use of chromium supplements should be reevaluated because the long-term biological effects of chromium accumulation in humans have not been determined.

Legal and Ethical Aspects

Chromium supplements are legal and ethical in conjunction with sport competition.

TABLE 8.11
Chromium Content of Common Foods in the Food Exchanges and Fast Foods

Meat/fish/poultry/cheese
1 ounce Canadian bacon = 4 micrograms
1 ounce smoked ham = 3 micrograms

Breads/cereals/legumes/starchy vegetables
1 cup dry oatmeal = 5 micrograms
1 cup shredded wheat cereals = 24 micrograms
4 graham crackers = 17 micrograms
1 cup baked beans = 140 micrograms

Vegetables
1 cup romaine lettuce = 16 micrograms
1 ounce green pepper = 5 micrograms

Fruits
1 banana = 18 micrograms
1/4 cantaloupe = 20 micrograms
4 ounces orange juice = 15 micrograms

Fast foods/snack foods/miscellaneous
1 McDonald's quarter-pound hamburger = 47 micrograms
1 ounce Doritos tortilla chips = 39 micrograms
1 cup brewed coffee = 21 micrograms

Source: G. A. Leville, M. E. Zabik, and K. J. Morgan. 1983. *Nutrients in Foods.* Cambridge, MA: The Nutrition Guild

Recommendations

Based on the available scientific evidence, chromium supplementation is not an effective sports ergogenic and its use is not recommended.

As with other trace minerals such as iron, some athletes might not obtain adequate chromium through their diets. Unfortunately, athletes cannot determine if they are chromium deficient because there is no reliable test to determine chromium status.

Athletes ideally should obtain adequate chromium through their diets, selecting foods rich in chromium as noted in table 8.11. If foods are not selected wisely, some athletes might benefit from chromium supplements, including (a) those who consume highly processed foods that have been depleted of chromium, (b) those who participate in weight-control sports and have inadequate chromium intake, (c) those who consume high-carbohydrate diets that may increase chromium needs, and (d) those who exercise strenuously because exercise increases chromium excretion in the urine. In such cases, the recommended procedure is to supplement the normal chromium intake with about 100–200 micrograms daily. The United States Olympic Committee indicates research does not support chromium intakes above the ESADDI.

Cocaine

Classification and Usage

Cocaine may be classified as a pharmacological sports ergogenic. Cocaine, an alkaloid derived from leaves of the coca plant, is a prescription drug used therapeutically as a topical anesthetic. Cocaine is a popular recreational drug with street names such as coke, snow, and crack, the latter being a more potent freebase form. Cocaine is inhaled into a nostril, smoked, or injected. Dosages used in human studies have approximated 4 to 5 grams.

Sports Performance Factor

Mental strength and physical power. Cocaine might be used primarily in attempts to enhance various sports performance factors that might benefit from a supplemental stimulant effect, and has been studied in attempts to enhance aerobic power and endurance.

Theory

Cocaine stimulates the central nervous system, including the sympathetic nervous system, inducing psychological feelings of exhilaration and decreased sensations of fatigue. Sympathetic nervous system physiological responses include increased heart rate and blood pressure. In general, it is theorized that the psychological and physiological effects of cocaine improve performance in a variety of sport endeavors by decreasing sensations of fatigue.

Effectiveness

Most research evaluating the ergogenic effect of cocaine has involved animals, including mice, rats, and horses. Physiological, metabolic, and performance tests have been conducted, the performance test normally being an exercise task to exhaustion. The results of animal studies are ambivalent, with studies showing either increases, decreases, or no change in exercise time to exhaustion.

Some anecdotal data suggest cocaine is an effective ergogenic, but controlled research studies with humans are almost nonexistent, probably because of the health risks noted below. Several studies in the early 1970s, using Andean native peoples who chewed coca leaves, reported no significant effect of cocaine on physiologic responses to exercise or on cycling time to exhaustion. The investigator noted, however, that performance time with cocaine was longer than with the placebo, and although statistically nonsignificant, he indicated this experimental finding was in accord with his empirical observations.

Although research is not supportive of an acute use of cocaine on sport performance, its role as a stimulant suggests it might, under some circumstances, be an effective sports ergogenic comparable to the use of other stimulants such as amphetamines and caffeine.

Safety

Cocaine is a highly addictive drug, and the Public Health Service recommends that individuals not even experiment with cocaine because a one-time use could lead to addiction.

Although the use of cocaine may lead to euphoria, acute cocaine use could be fatal as documented by heart attacks in several prominent young athletes. Cocaine stimulates the heart, but at the same time decreases blood flow to the heart muscle, a situation that can induce ventricular fibrillation (very rapid, inefficient heartbeats) and subsequent heart failure.

Chronic cocaine use may also contribute to a series of health problems, including liver toxicity, cerebrovascular stroke, and symptoms of mental illness. Use of needles to inject cocaine increases risk of hepatitis and HIV infection.

Legal and Ethical Aspects

Cocaine use as a sports ergogenic is prohibited by most athletic governing bodies and is considered unethical behavior. Cocaine use by athletes as a recreational drug is prohibited by many athletic governing bodies. Cocaine distribution and use is illegal and subject to criminal penalties.

Recommendations

Cocaine use is not recommended as a sports ergogenic because it is illegal, unethical, and may be associated with serious health risks. Although the theory underlying cocaine use as a sports ergogenic is persuasive, there are insufficient data to support its effectiveness for improving sports performance. Some data suggest acute cocaine use might impair performance.

> I think it [cocaine] slowed me down, not only running but mental things too.
>
> —Lonnie Smith, Kansas City Royals

Coenzyme Q$_{10}$ (CoQ$_{10}$, Ubiquinone)

Classification and Usage

Coenzyme Q$_{10}$, also known as CoQ$_{10}$ and ubiquinone, is a dietary supplement that may be classified as a nutritional sports ergogenic. CoQ$_{10}$ supplements are available in pill and capsule extract form, either individually or in combination with other purported nutritional ergogenics such as inosine and vitamin E.

Researchers have used dosages ranging from 100 to 150 milligrams per day for several months.

Sports Performance Factor

Physical power. CoQ$_{10}$ supplementation has been studied in attempts to increase aerobic power and endurance for sport events that derive energy primarily from the oxygen energy system.

Theory

CoQ$_{10}$ is involved in several metabolic processes in the human body that may be important for the optimal functioning of the oxygen energy system. CoQ$_{10}$ is found in the mitochondria of all tissues and is an important component of the electron transport system that generates ATP via oxidative processes. CoQ$_{10}$ is an antioxidant that may help prevent cellular damage from oxygen free radicals generated during intense aerobic exercise.

Because research has found that CoQ$_{10}$ supplementation improved heart function, V̇O$_2$max, and exercise performance in cardiac patients, CoQ$_{10}$ advocates theorized it could be an effective sports ergogenic for healthy aerobic endurance athletes.

Effectiveness

Although some studies included in a book detailing the clinical uses of CoQ$_{10}$ suggested it was an effective sports ergogenic, these studies suffered from one or more methodological flaws, such as no control group or no placebo, and have not been published in peer-reviewed, scientific journals.

Studies published in scientific journals do not support the effectiveness of CoQ$_{10}$ supplementation as a sports ergogenic, either taken separately or as part of a commercial product containing other alleged nutritional ergogenics. Such supplementation has not been shown to prevent lipid peroxidation during exercise or to enhance metabolic responses to either submaximal or maximal exercise, the anaerobic or lactate threshold, V̇O$_2$max, or cycle ergometer exercise time to exhaustion in either young or old athletes. Moreover, in a recent anaerobic exercise training study from Sweden, subjects taking the placebo improved their anaerobic performance on repetitive 10-second all-out cycling tests, whereas subjects taking CoQ$_{10}$ supplements for 20 days showed no improvement. Thus, well-controlled research does not support the effectiveness of CoQ$_{10}$ supplementation as a sports ergogenic, and suggests supplementation may impair performance in anaerobic exercise tasks.

Safety

CoQ$_{10}$ supplementation in doses of 100 to 150 milligrams for several months appears to be safe. No adverse effects were noted in most studies that used these dosages. However, in the Swedish study cited above, subjects who supplemented with 120 milligrams of CoQ$_{10}$ daily for 20 days showed evidence of muscle tissue damage compared to subjects taking the placebo. The authors speculate this may actually be due to a pro-oxidant effect and increased damage from free radicals. The authors also suggest this was the reason anaerobic performance did not improve compared to the subjects taking the placebo.

Legal and Ethical Aspects

CoQ_{10} supplementation is legal and ethical in conjunction with sport competition.

Recommendations

Based on available scientific evidence (although additional research is desirable), the contemporary viewpoint is that CoQ_{10} supplementation is not an effective sports ergogenic and its use is not recommended.

Creatine

Classification and Usage.

Creatine may be classified as a physiological sports ergogenic, but some may regard it as a nutritional sports ergogenic. Creatine is an amine, a natural dietary constituent present in small amounts in animal foods, but it also may be synthesized in the liver and kidney from several amino acids.

Most studies involving the ergogenic effect of creatine supplementation used doses approximating 20–30 grams per day, consumed in 4–5 equal doses throughout the day, for 5–7 days. The most common form used was creatine monohydrate powder consumed with fluids. Many athletic teams in the United States supplement with creatine. Figure 8.12 displays one brand of creatine supplement.

Sports Performance Factor

Physical power and mechanical edge. Creatine supplementation is used in attempts to increase high power and speed in sport events that derive energy primarily from the ATP-CP energy system. Creatine supplementation also has been studied in relation to increased body mass.

Theory

The normal daily requirement of dietary and endogenously synthesized creatine approximates 2 grams, an amount that is adequate for generating normal intramuscular creatine phosphate (CP) levels.

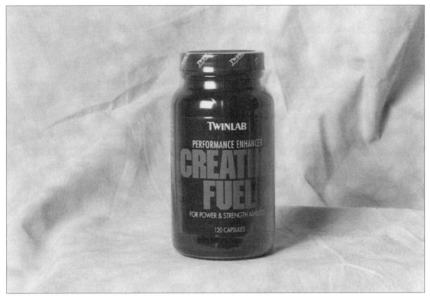

Figure 8.12 Creatine supplements are popular with strength-trained athletes.

Creatine supplementation could increase the whole body creatine pool, theoretically facilitating the generation of CP. Muscle stores of CP may split and release energy for the rapid resynthesis of ATP, although the supply of CP, like that of ATP, is limited. The combined total of ATP and CP might sustain maximal energy production for approximately 5–10 seconds of maximal effort, and thus would be the primary energy source in dash events ranging from 50–100 meters. Fatigue in such events may be attributed to the rapid decrease in CP. Thus, a more rapid recovery of CP would enhance ATP formation and improve performance in sports demanding high power and speed.

Effectiveness

Several studies have shown that oral creatine supplementation in amounts approximating 20–30 grams per day for 5 to 7 days significantly increased intramuscular concentrations of both free creatine and CP during rest and during recovery after intense exercise. Some subjects, however, were nonresponders, as their muscle CP levels did not increase. Vegetarians, who have limited dietary creatine intake, would benefit most from creatine supplementation. Consuming creatine with glucose may enhance creatine uptake into the body.

Several dozen recent well-controlled laboratory and field studies have investigated the ergogenic effects of creatine supplementation on exercise tasks associated with the ATP-CP energy system, but the findings are equivocal. Some studies found that creatine supplementation improved performance in the later stages of repetitive, short-term (4–10 seconds), high-intensity cycle ergometer sprint tests, while others revealed significant increases in muscle force during repetitive bouts of isotonic, isometric, and isokinetic resistance testing. Research findings from studies investigating the effects of creatine supplementation on single bouts of high-intensity exercise are less supportive. Additionally, well-controlled field studies involving the effect of creatine supplementation on repeat 60-meter run sprints and 25-meter or 50-meter swim sprints reveal no ergogenic effect.

Some research suggests creatine supplementation may serve as a buffer in the muscle and may decrease muscle lactate accumulation, enhancing performance in sport events dependent on the lactic acid energy system. Available research findings are too few and clearly equivocal. Relative to performance, one study found that creatine supplementation improved rowing performance in a 1,000-meter race by 2.3 seconds. Other studies reported no significant effect on either a 100-meter swim test or anaerobic cycle tests at supramaximal levels (115–125 percent of VO_2 max) designed to stress the lactic acid energy system. More research is needed to clarify these ambiguous data.

Creatine supplementation might be detrimental to performance in events dependent primarily on the oxygen energy system. Creatine phosphate is not a very important energy source for prolonged aerobic exercise, and one of the side effects of creatine supplementation, an increased body mass, has been suggested as a detrimental effect of creatine supplementation on performance in a 6-kilometer run over undulating terrain. It would cost more energy to move the additional body weight.

One consistent finding in most studies is an increased body mass. A week of creatine supplementation has been found to increase body mass by about .9–2.2 kilograms (2.0–4.6 pounds). It is not evident that the increased body mass is lean muscle tissue, but, given the rapidity of the weight gain, most likely is water weight bound to creatine. Some research has noted a decrease in urine production associated with creatine supplementation, which is an indirect marker of fluid retention in the body.

If, however, creatine supplementation enhances resistance training over time, the result may be an increased muscle mass, or lean body mass, and associated gains in strength and power.

Several recent reviews have suggested creatine supplementation may be an effective sport ergogenic. This may be true, but as noted, the ergogenic effect may be specific to certain types of performance, i.e., repetitive, high-intensity, very short-term exercise tasks with brief recovery periods. It also is possible that creatine supplementation enables an athlete to engage in more intense physical training, which eventually could translate into enhanced sports performance. Well-controlled laboratory and field research is needed to document the potential of creatine supplementation as an effective sport ergogenic.

> **C**reatine should not be viewed as another gimmick supplement; its ingestion is a means of providing immediate, significant performance improvements to athletes involved in explosive sports.
> —*Paul Greenhaff, British exercise physiologist*

Safety

Creatine supplementation appears to pose no acute health risks, insofar as there are no reports of adverse effects in studies investigating its ergogenic potential. Health risks associated with long-term supplementation have not been determined. Some anecdotal information indicates creatine supplementation might cause muscle cramping, possibly due to the increased muscle water content diluting electrolyte levels.

Legal and Ethical Aspects

Creatine is currently legal for use by athletes. Creatine supplementation may contravene the general meaning of the International Olympic Committee anti-doping legislation; i.e., consuming a substance in abnormal quantities with the intent of artificially and unfairly enhancing sports performance. Depending on the athlete's viewpoint, creatine supplementation may be ethical or unethical.

Recommendations

Creatine supplementation may be an effective sports ergogenic for specific exercise tasks dependent on the ATP-CP energy system, particularly repetitive, high-power tasks with brief recovery periods. Creatine use may enable sprint-type athletes to recover more rapidly in training and thus its use may increase training intensity.

If you decide to experiment with creatine supplementation, about 20 grams per day (4 doses of 5 grams each consumed over the day) should increase your muscle creatine levels within 5 to 7 days. To enhance the storage of creatine in the muscles, consume 90 grams of carbohydrates with each 5-gram dose. A slower technique would be to consume 3 grams of creatine a day for about 1 month. Two grams per day will maintain muscle creatine levels once they are full.

However, creatine supplementation would not be recommended for aerobic endurance sport competition because increased body mass could impair performance. Creatine appears to be safe if consumed in appropriate amounts, and is legal. Whether its use is ethical or not is debatable. The decision to use creatine in attempts to enhance sports performance is up to the individual athlete.

DHEA (Dehydroepiandrosterone)

Classification and Usage

Dehydroepiandrosterone (DHEA), or its ester *dehydroepiandrosterone sulfate (DHEA-S)*, may be classified as a physiological sports ergogenic because it is a natural steroid hormone produced endogenously by the adrenal gland. DHEA also may be classified as a nutritional sports ergogenic because some forms, including pure DHEA or herbal precursors that are advertised to be converted to DHEA in the body, are marketed as dietary supplements. Human studies normally use ranges from 50 to 100 milligrams per day, but some research has used doses as high as 1,600 milligrams daily. DHEA may be taken orally or injected.

Sports Performance Factor

Mechanical edge and physical power. DHEA is used primarily to increase muscle mass and decrease body fat for enhanced strength and power or for a more aesthetic physical appearance in sports such as bodybuilding.

Theory

Although the functions of DHEA in the human body are unknown, it may be converted into other hormones, particularly testosterone and estrogen. Some research indicates DHEA supplementation may increase serum levels of insulin-like growth factor I (IGF-I), an anabolic substance associated with human growth hormone secretion. Given its potential effect on testosterone and IGF-I, DHEA supplementation is theorized to stimulate anabolic activity, increasing muscle mass and decreasing body fat.

Effectiveness

Animal research suggests that DHEA supplementation may decrease the incidence of several chronic diseases, including obesity, by decreasing fat and increasing muscle mass. Most animal studies, however, involved rodents which have little natural DHEA. In humans, natural DHEA production is high during young adulthood and begins to diminish at age 30 and beyond, possibly reaching very low levels at age 50 and beyond, although individual values may vary substantially. Much of the research with humans has focused on older subjects, those aged 50 and over, who might benefit from DHEA replenishment.

There are limited data substantiating the effectiveness of DHEA supplementation as a sports ergogenic. In one study, DHEA supplementation (100 milligrams per day for 3 months) decreased body fat and increased lean muscle mass and strength in both men and women aged 50 to 65, but the subjects were sedentary. Other research has indicated improvements in perceived physical and psychological well-being, but no exercise tasks were studied. Conversely, other studies have not shown any beneficial effects of DHEA supplementation on body composition in sedentary, older subjects.

One writer notes that DHEA supplementation may benefit young endurance athletes who might have low serum testosterone levels due to extensive training, but no research data are available to support this contention.

Safety

DHEA supplementation is being studied clinically because some medical investigators believe it may help prevent several chronic diseases, including heart disease, diabetes, and cancer. Most human studies involving DHEA supplementation have not reported any major adverse side effects, but some abnormal findings have occurred, including an increase in facial hair and decreased levels of HDL cholesterol (the good cholesterol) in women, presumably due to effects of testosterone. Additionally, although future research may support some health benefits of DHEA supplementation, most scientists recommend caution, and suggest no one should take DHEA unless under the supervision of a physician. A recent review of DHEA supplementation and aging by the publishers of *The New England Journal of Medicine* indicated that there are no proven benefits and some potentially serious risks. The long-term effects of DHEA supplementation are not known, but two possible effects include liver toxicity and prostate cancer in males.

Legal and Ethical Aspects

Use of DHEA is prohibited by the International Olympic Committee. It is a corticosteroid that could stimulate testosterone production, and thus may possess anabolic properties. Its use would be illegal and unethical.

Recommendations

There are insufficient data to support the effectiveness of DHEA supplementation as a sports ergogenic, and thus its use cannot be recommended at this time, particularly with young, healthy athletes. Medical authorities indicate DHEA supplementation may pose some serious health risks, so safety concerns also discourage recommendation of DHEA. Moreover, DHEA is illegal and unethical because its use has been prohibited by the IOC.

Diuretics

Classification and Usage

Diuretics may be classified as a pharmacological sports ergogenic. Diuretics represent a class of drugs that are used therapeutically to increase the secretion of urine and to eliminate excess body water under certain pathological conditions, including the treatment of high blood pressure. Numerous types of diuretics are available, as listed in appendix A. The dosage depends on the type of diuretic used.

Sports Performance Factor

Mechanical edge. Diuretics have been studied in attempts to provide a mechanical edge to some athletes, indirectly enhancing the efficiency of energy production, particularly the ATP-CP and lactic acid energy systems, per unit body weight.

Theory

Athletes in weight-control sports such as boxing, wrestling, and weightlifting may use diuretics to lose weight rapidly in order to qualify for particular weight classes in competition. Gymnasts, high jumpers, and athletes in other sports in which excess body weight might be a disadvantage also might use diuretics. Diuretics may induce a 3 percent or greater reduction in body mass within a relatively short period of time. For a 160-pound athlete, this would be approximately 5 pounds. If these body water losses do not impair performance, then the wrestler in a lower weight class, the gymnast with less weight to support on the rings, and the high jumper with a few pounds less to get over the bar may have a competitive advantage because of a higher ratio of power production to body weight (figure 8.13). Sir Isaac Newton's second law of motion states that acceleration is proportional to force production and inversely proportional to mass; therefore, decreasing mass and keeping force constant results in greater acceleration.

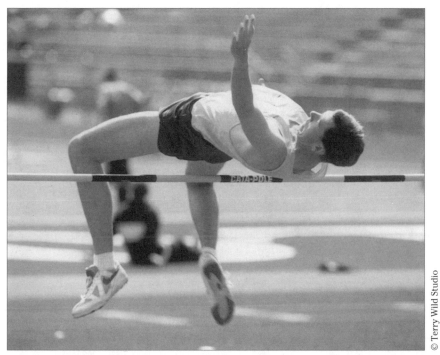

© Terry Wild Studio

Figure 8.13 Diuretics may help athletes lose body water rapidly without losing muscle power, increasing the possibility of their lifting lower masses to greater heights.

Athletes also have used diuretics, not for a direct ergogenic effect, but to avoid detection of the use of illegal pharmacological sports ergogenics. Because of their ability to increase urine production and secretion, some diuretics also increase the excretion rate of certain prohibited agents and their metabolites. Some athletes hope the use of diuretics will help them to excrete the prohibited drug prior to the urine test that determines drug use, although sophisticated drug testing for both diuretics and other drugs is deterring the use of diuretics for this purpose.

Effectiveness

Based on the laws of physics, it is logical to assume that a wrestler, gymnast, or high jumper is at a competitive advantage at a lower weight, provided energy production is not diminished. Although little evidence documents a direct improvement in sports performance following the use of diuretics, some recent data suggest beneficial effects.

In general, research has shown that diuretics may lead to substantial body water losses, more than 3 percent, and not result in any deterioration in strength, power, or local muscular endurance of an anaerobic nature. Thus, in sports characterized by brief, intense effort, performance seemingly would not be compromised by use of diuretic agents and may be benefited. Research has revealed, for example, that the use of a diuretic to lose weight leads to improvement in vertical jumping ability.

Conversely, use of diuretics might impair aerobic endurance capacity. Diuretics may produce an 8 to 10 percent decrease in plasma volume even though body weight loss is only 3 percent. This plasma volume decrease has resulted in impaired cardiovascular functions during exercise, such as a decrease in the amount of blood pumped per heartbeat. In runners, the use of diuretics has been shown to slow performance by 8 seconds in a 1.5-kilometer race, 78 seconds in a 5-kilometer race, and 157 seconds in a 10-kilometer race.

Diuretics may be an effective ergogenic for certain sports, but may be ergolytic and impair performance in others.

Safety

Dizziness, a common side effect of diuretics, could impair motor control in all athletes. Diuretic-induced dehydration could lead to serious health problems for athletes training or competing in warm temperatures, because those athletes are more susceptible to heat exhaustion or heatstroke. Some diuretics excrete electrolytes such as potassium. Thus, the chronic use of diuretics can lead to low levels of body potassium and disturbed neurological functioning, with symptoms ranging from muscular weakness and cramps to disturbances of normal heart function.

Legal and Ethical Aspects

Diuretics are prohibited by the International Olympic Committee. The use of diuretics as a sports ergogenic is illegal and unethical.

Recommendations

Although diuretics may be an effective sports ergogenic for certain athletes, diuretic use is not recommended because it is illegal and unethical. Athletes should reach an acceptable body weight and maintain optimal energy production through proper diet and exercise programs. Nondrug techniques are available for reducing excess body water prior to competition, although practices such as sauna-induced dehydration are denounced by several professional sports medicine organizations.

Engineered Dietary Supplements

Classification and Usage

Engineered dietary supplements, sometimes referred to as engineered foods, may be classified as a nutritional sports ergogenic. These supplements are the result of advances in nutritional biotechnology that permit the isolation of specific nutrients, metabolic byproducts, or other substances with alleged sports ergogenic potential. Some engineered dietary supplements such as HMB (beta-hydroxy-beta-methylbutyrate) contain a single substance. Others, such as Hot Stuff, contain a blend of more than 30 ingredients ranging from boron to transferulic acid, while still others such as MET-Rx contain special ingredients such as Metamyosyn, purportedly not found in any other product.

A recent survey of advertising for nutritional supplements in health and bodybuilding magazines revealed 89 brands, 311 products, and 235 unique ingredients. The most frequently promoted benefit was muscle growth.

Numerous commercially engineered dietary supplements are targeted for the athlete or the physically active person, mostly for those wanting to lose body fat and gain muscle mass. Recommended dosages vary depending on the brand.

Sports Performance Factor

Mechanical edge and physical power. Most engineered dietary supplements are advertised primarily as anabolic agents for increasing muscle mass and decrease body fat for enhanced strength and power or for a more aesthetic physical appearance in sports such as bodybuilding. Other products may be developed for aerobic endurance athletes.

Theory

There may be as many theories regarding anabolic effects as there are ingredients in these products. For example: (a) HMB, a metabolic byproduct of the amino acid leucine, is alleged to retard the breakdown of muscle protein during strenuous resistance exercise; (b) boron and transferulic acid are theorized to enhance the secretion of the anabolic hormone testosterone; and (c) Metamyosyn is a complex

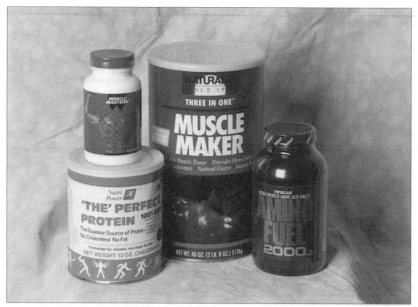

Figure 8.14 Numerous engineered dietary supplements appear on the market every year, many targeted to physically active individuals and athletes.

of 50 protein isolates theorized to help MET-Rx burn fat and build muscle (figure 8.14).

Effectiveness

In most cases, advertisements suggesting that engineered dietary supplements are powerful anabolic agents are not based on scientific evidence, but rather on theory and anecdotal evidence from athletes, who usually are paid to endorse the product.

In general, companies that market engineered foods or dietary supplements do not provide funding for independent research to evaluate the product's effectiveness. For example, there appear to be no scientific data specifically evaluating the effectiveness of MET-Rx. One study provided some indirect evidence indicating that MET-Rx is not an effective sports ergogenic. In this study, investigators were evaluating the effectiveness of another purported nutritional sports ergogenic (HMB) and were interested in the possible interaction effect of protein. Their research design consisted of six groups of subjects undergoing 3 weeks of resistance strength training; two of the groups did not consume any HMB, but one group received a protein supplement, which was MET-Rx, and the other group did not. There were no significant differences between these two groups for body composition or strength changes, suggesting MET-Rx was not an effective sports ergogenic when added to a diet that already contained a normal dietary intake of protein, which in this study was about twice the recommended dietary allowance.

Some products may be effective ergogenics if they contain substances, such as creatine, that have been shown by some well-controlled research to increase body weight and strength. Other substances such as HMB may be shown to be effective anabolics in the future. Animal studies have indicated HMB supplementation may increase lean muscle mass and decrease body fat, and some preliminary findings with humans are supportive.

Safety

Many engineered dietary supplements lack appropriate safety data. Those that primarily contain nutrients are unlikely to be harmful unless consumed in excess. For example, MET-Rx contains primarily milk-based protein, carbohydrate, fat, vitamins, minerals, and other natural nutrients found in foods we eat. Some preparations, however, may cause health problems, particularly herbal ingredients that could evoke anaphylactic reactions in some people.

Legal and Ethical Aspects

Use of engineered dietary supplements as a sports ergogenic is legal and ethical, provided they contain no prohibited ingredients.

Recommendations

In general, engineered dietary supplements are not recommended as a sports ergogenic because very few of these products have been studied adequately in order to substantiate advertised claims.

Literature accompanying the sale of these products should contain references to studies published in reputable scientific journals. You may check out the validity of this research by calling the Gatorade Sport Science Institute, 800-616-4774, or the Food Nutrition Information Center at the National Agriculture Library, 301-504-5719.

Ephedrine (Sympathomimetics)

Classification and Usage

Ephedrine, a synthetic sympathomimetic drug, may be classified as a pharmacological sports ergogenic. Other sympathomimetic drugs include pseudoephedrine and phenylephrine. Sympathomimetic drugs are designed to mimic the effects of the natural, endogenous hormones norepinephrine (noradrenalin) and epinephrine (adrenaline), eliciting physiologic responses from the sympathetic nervous system. Sympathomimetic drugs may be selective (eliciting specific physiologic effects) or nonselective (eliciting a general sympathetic response). Ephedrine, a nonselective sympathomimetic, may be used therapeutically for various health problems, including treatment of asthma and symptoms of the common cold. Ephedrine also may be used to promote weight loss.

Ephedrine or other sympathomimetics are found in various antiasthmatic and cold or cough medications in either pill, tablet, or inhaler form, including Primatene, Bronkotabs, Co-Tylenol, Vicks Inhaler, and Alka-Seltzer Plus (figure 8.15). Ephedrine also is found in herbal teas and dietary supplements containing Ma Huang (Chinese Ephedra or herbal ephedrine) as well as in dietary supplements marketed for weight loss and for increasing energy. All cold medications with decongestants are likely to contain prohibited sympathomimetics. See appendix A for a more extensive list.

The dose of ephedrine or other sympathomimetics varies with the product used. Inhalers usually provide a more rapid response. Doses

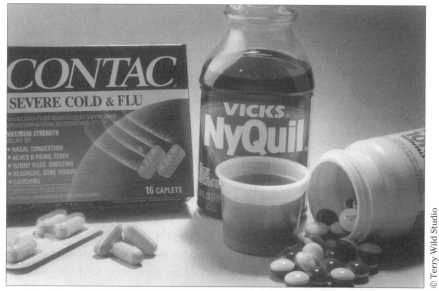

Figure 8.15 Many over-the-counter medications contain ephedrine, a drug that is is prohibited for use by athletes.

used in research approximate 20 to 25 milligrams of ephedrine (a full therapeutic dose) and 120 milligrams of pseudoephedrine. Check over-the-counter medications for ephedrine content.

Sports Performance Factor

Mental strength and physical power. Ephedrine and other sympathomimetics may be used in attempts to enhance various sports performance factors that may benefit from a supplemental stimulant effect, including physical power from all three human energy systems, the ATP-CP, lactic acid, and oxygen energy systems. Some athletes may use ephedrine to curb the appetite for weight loss and a possible mechanical edge.

Theory

By activating the sympathetic response, ephedrine may enhance muscle contractility, increase the blood output of the heart, enlarge the bronchial pathways to the lungs, and increase blood sugar levels. Theoretically, this sympathetic response could enhance all types of physical power, most notably aerobic endurance performance.

Effectiveness

Although limited, the available research does not support a sports ergogenic effect of sympathomimetics. In one study, a full therapeutic oral dose of ephedrine did not improve metabolic, psychological, or performance responses in tests of strength, power, muscular endurance, reaction time, speed, anaerobic capacity, or aerobic endurance capacity. Another study has shown that pseudoephedrine had no effect on muscular strength or on a 40-kilometer time trial in trained cyclists, with nearly identical times of 58 minutes under pseudoephedrine and placebo conditions.

Safety

Use of ephedrine or other sympathomimetics may elicit side effects, such as nervous tension, headache, gastrointestinal distress, and irregular heartbeats. Some individuals might suffer seizures and psychoses. In the United States, the Food and Drug Administration has received reports documenting numerous adverse health episodes, including at least 17 deaths, associated with use of ephedrine-containing products and is currently planning to restrict its use in dietary supplements and possibly including a label warning that use of this product may cause death.

Legal and Ethical Aspects

Use of ephedrine and other sympathomimetics as stimulants is prohibited by the International Olympic Committee. Some sports governing bodies, however, have not prohibited or do not test for ephedrine and similar sympathomimetics. Athletes need to check with their specific organizations regarding legality. If prohibited, use of these agents would be unethical. Some investigators are lobbying to have the IOC ban repealed, as no research supports an ergogenic effect of the sympathomimetics used in the treatment of asthma or cold symptoms. The list may be found in appendix A.

In the 1972 Munich Olympics, Rick DeMont won a gold medal in swimming, but was disqualified because he tested positive for ephedrine. Being asthmatic, DeMont was taking a medication that contained ephedrine.

Recommendations

The use of ephedrine or other sympathomimetics as sports ergogenics is not recommended because no research has supported their effectiveness for enhancing performance and their use may be associated with some severe health risks. Their use in some sport events is illegal and unethical. Athletes who use medications containing these drugs should consult with their respective sport governing bodies to determine whether their use is legal. Legal anti-asthmatic medications are listed in appendix A.

In the 1996 Olympics, at least six athletes tested positive for drug use, mostly stimulants obtained from over-the-counter products.

Erythropoietin (EPO, rEPO)

Classification and Usage

Erythropoietin (EPO) may be considered a physiological sports ergogenic. EPO is a natural hormone secreted by the kidney. EPO stimulates the formation of red blood cells (RBCs) in the bone marrow. Through genetic engineering, a synthetic form (rEPO) has been developed using recombinant technology. Technically, rEPO may be classified as a drug, or a pharmacological sports ergogenic. Some anecdotal information indicates use of rEPO by aerobic endurance athletes. Dosages in research with healthy males approximated 20–40 IU rEPO per kilogram body weight three times a week for 6 weeks. rEPO is administered by injection either intravenously or subcutaneously.

Sports Performance Factor

Physical power. The synthetic hormone rEPO is used in attempts to increase aerobic power and endurance in sport events that derive energy primarily from the oxygen energy system.

Theory

rEPO is designed to stimulate the production of RBCs in the bone marrow and, comparable to blood doping, increase the concentration of RBCs and hemoglobin in the blood (figure 8.16). The hemoglobin in the RBC binds with oxygen in the lungs for transport to the muscle; thus the increased oxygen-carrying capacity of the blood may provide an ergogenic effect for sports involving the oxygen energy system—aerobic power and endurance events over 5 minutes.

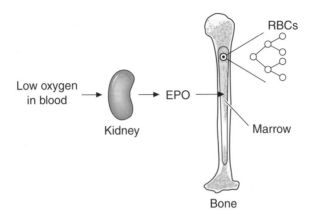

Figure 8.16 Low oxygen levels in the blood stimulate the release of erythropoietin from the kidney. EPO travels to the bone marrow and stimulates the development of red blood cells.

Effectiveness

rEPO injections have been shown to increase RBC production and hemoglobin concentration in the blood from 6–11 percent over 6 weeks. Although fewer studies are available compared to blood doping research, EPO injections have been shown to increase VO_2max and endurance performance as measured by treadmill run time to exhaustion. In a recent review, the American College of Sports Medicine indicated that EPO administration in healthy subjects seems to provide ergogenic effects similar to those seen with blood doping. Thus, like blood doping, rEPO is a very potent sports ergogenic.

Safety

Injections of rEPO could pose health risks even with medical supervision, and these risks may increase if athletes are medically unsupervised. Health risks associated with EPO administration include infections (hepatitis B, HIV) from use of contaminated needles, increased resting and exercise blood pressure, increased hematocrit, increased blood viscosity, thrombosis, and even myocardial infarction. Unsupervised EPO use has been suggested as a link to the deaths of more than a few young elite cyclists. Some experts refer to rEPO as the drug used by athletes who live by the motto: "Better dead than second."

Legal and Ethical Aspects

The use of rEPO as a sports ergogenic is illegal and unethical. The IOC lists it as a prohibited substance. Current urine drug testing tech-

> The recent death of another young Dutch cyclist makes a total of four such deaths in the past two years…there has been widespread speculation that they may be related to the use of a synthetic form of the hormone erythropoietin (EPO).
>
> —J. E. Ramotar, writer for Physician and Sportsmedicine

niques may detect rEPO use for only 2–3 days following the last administration; however, the physiological effects of rEPO may last for weeks, making the drug test moot. Thus, the International Cycling Union has initiated blood tests and has banned athletes with hematocrits (percentage of red blood cells) greater than 50 from competition. The American College of Sports Medicine, an international organization, declared the use of rEPO to improve athletic performance unethical.

Recommendations

Although rEPO is a very effective sports ergogenic and may be safe to use with proper medical precautions, its use has been prohibited and therefore is not recommended.

A male athlete was expelled from the Olympic village in the 1996 Atlanta Olympic games after admitting to using rEPO.

Another viable, legal, and ethical method may be available, however. Some athletes have attempted to increase RBC concentration by living and training at high altitudes, approximately 2,000 meters or 6,500 feet above sea level. The low oxygen pressure stimulates the release of EPO from the kidney, leading to an increased RBC concentration. However, the low oxygen pressure also appears to decrease training intensity, possibly counterbalancing the benefits from increased RBC concentration. Thus, performance normally has not been shown to improve upon return to sea level.

Several investigators have reported recently that living at altitude and training at sea level provides the best of both worlds. Living at altitude stimulates increases in RBC, while training at sea level permits optimal high-intensity exercise. Living high and training low may not be practical for most athletes, given geographical and travel constraints. It is, however, possible in many countries. Moreover, special high-altitude houses to maintain low oxygen levels comparable to 2,000 meters or more have been developed at sea level. The athlete can live and sleep in a low-oxygen environment to stimulate RBC production, and walk out the door to train at sea level. Preliminary research suggests that living high and training low may enhance performance not only in aerobic endurance events, but also in anaerobic endurance events.

Fat Supplementation

Classification and Usage

Fat supplements may be classified as a nutritional sports ergogenic. Dietary fats are found naturally in many foods we eat, mainly in animal foods such as meat and milk, but also in varying amounts in plant foods, low in most fruits and vegetables and rather high in nuts and seeds. The fats we eat are known as triglycerides, combinations of free fatty acids (FFA) and glycerol. Some fat is needed in the diet because it provides us with several essential fatty acids and fat-soluble vitamins. No Recommended Dietary Allowance (RDA) has been established for total fat, but the National Research Council indicates we need about 3–6 grams of essential fatty acids, which is readily obtainable even on a vegetarian diet containing only about 5 to 10 percent of dietary calories as fat.

One of the major functions of fat in the human body is to provide energy, as discussed previously.

Various commercial fat supplements are marketed to athletes, primarily medium-chain triglycerides (MCTs). MCTs are sold in liquid form and also are incorporated in some sport drinks and sport bars. Infusions of triglyceride emulsions have been studied in attempts to enhance sports performance.

Sports Performance Factor

Physical power. Fat supplementation is used in attempts to increase aerobic endurance for sport events that derive energy primarily from the oxygen energy system.

Theory

The preferred fuel for high-intensity aerobic exercise is carbohydrate, but the liver and muscles have a limited capacity to store carbohydrate in the form of glycogen and may become depleted in very prolonged athletic events—in running events of more than 20 miles, for example. Fat also is an energy source for aerobic exercise, so it may be advantageous for some endurance athletes to optimize fat utilization as an energy source in order to spare enough liver and muscle glycogen for the later stages of an aerobic endurance contest.

Because the rate of FFA oxidation in the muscle is partly dependent on the FFA concentration in the blood, various fat supplementation techniques have been used in attempts to increase blood FFA: (a) low-carbohydrate–high-fat diets are designed to provide more dietary fats, which could increase blood FFA following digestion, absorption, and processing by the liver; (b) infusion of triglyceride emulsions may increase blood FFA after processing by the liver; and (c) ingestion of MCTs, which are absorbed rapidly because they are water soluble, are processed by the liver to form FFA that may be converted into ketones, which may pass into the blood and serve as another energy source for the muscle during exercise.

Effectiveness

Although a low carbohydrate-high fat diet may increase the utilization of fat as an energy source during exercise, no reputable scientific data indicate such a diet will enhance high-intensity, aerobic endurance performance when compared to a high-carbohydrate diet or a mixed diet. Conversely, low-carbohydrate, high-fat diets may actually impair performance because of inadequate carbohydrate, the primary energy source during such exercise. It should be noted that athletes might train quite effectively with a diet of from 30 percent to 40 percent fat calories, particularly if they consume a high-calorie diet. An athlete who consumes 3,600 calories per day, 50 percent being derived from carbohydrate, will receive 450 grams of carbohydrate, a rather substantial amount.

Some research suggests that infusion of triglyceride emulsions will elevate FFA in the blood and possibly spare muscle glycogen utilization, but studies have not reported significant improvements in physical performance.

Several studies have shown that ingested MCTs may be oxidized during exercise, but will not spare the use of muscle glycogen and have not been shown to enhance physical performance. Several studies have evaluated the effects of a combined MCT-carbohydrate supplement, and although the findings conflict, one study did reveal an ergogenic effect. In three different trials, cyclists consumed either a carbohydrate solution, an MCT solution, or a combined MCT-carbohydrate solution. They exercised at 60 percent of $\dot{V}O_2$max for 2 hours, and then completed a 40-kilometer time trial. Performance in the 40-kilometer ride was worst with the MCT trial, but the MCT-carbohydrate trial produced the fastest time, which the investigators attributed to a sparing of muscle glycogen during the 2-hour ride. This is an interesting finding, but additional research is needed to confirm it.

Safety

Although fat supplementation techniques may be safe if used in moderation, each carries some health risks. A chronic low-carbohydrate, high-fat diet might predispose individuals to heart disease and colon cancer. Infused triglyceride emulsions, if not carefully controlled, might lead to excess FFA concentration in the blood. Ingestion of MCT in amounts greater than 30 grams have been associated with gastrointestinal distress and diarrhea.

Legal and Ethical Aspects

Low-carbohydrate, high-fat diets and ingestion of MCTs are legal and ethical in conjunction with sport competition. However, infusion of triglyceride emulsions may contravene the general meaning of the International Olympic Committee anti-doping legislation, i.e., taking a substance by an abnormal route of entry with the intent of artificially and unfairly enhancing sports performance. Hence, its use may be unethical.

Recommendations

Based on available scientific evidence, fat supplementation is not an effective sports ergogenic for most athletes, and its use is not recommended. Diets high in fat will not improve but may actually impair an athlete's performance and long-term health, while triglyceride emulsion infusions also do not enhance performance and might carry significant health risks.

Compared to carbohydrate ingestion, ingestion of MCTs might impair performance. However, one study suggests that consumption of an MCT-carbohydrate supplement may improve performance more than a carbohydrate supplement. Although more research is needed to confirm this finding and to determine optimal concentrations, this study used a sport drink mixture containing 10 percent carbohydrate and about a 4 percent MCT concentration. Such a solution may be concocted by purchasing MCTs at a health food store and adding 40 grams to a liter (1,000 milliliters) of a 10 percent carbohydrate sport drink. About 400 milliliters (about 13.5 ounces) should be consumed before and 100 milliliters (about 3.5 ounces) every 10 minutes during exercise.

Various agents have been used in attempts to mobilize FFA during exercise so that they might be used preferentially as a fuel and therefore help spare the utilization of muscle glycogen. In this regard, caffeine may be effective (see Caffeine).

Fluid Supplementation (Sport Drinks)

Classification and Usage

Fluid supplementation may be classified as a nutritional sports ergogenic. Water, our most essential nutrient, is the major fluid supplement. Other fluid supplements such as fruit juices, sodas, and sport drinks are mostly water, but may contain other nutrients or dietary constituents such as carbohydrate, electrolytes, vitamins, minerals, choline, and glycerol.

Water may be obtained directly from the tap or from bottled sources. Numerous varieties of other fluid replacements, such as sport drinks, are commercially available.

Sport drinks used to contain only water, sugar, and some electrolytes. Now they may contain more exotic substances alleged to be ergogenic, such as choline and glycerol.

Sports Performance Factor

Physical power. Fluid supplementation is used in attempts to enhance aerobic power and endurance performance, particularly under warm environmental conditions.

Theory

Your body is approximately 60 percent water, and water is the environment within which all of your other nutrients function. Dehydration, or the loss of body water, can disturb cardiovascular function, cell metabolism, and temperature regulation. In general, dehydration leading to body weight losses of only 2 percent may lead to decreases in aerobic endurance capacity. The greater the fluid loss, the more performance suffers. For a 150-pound runner, a loss of 3 pounds represents a 2 percent dehydration. In a hot environment, such a loss can occur in less than 30 minutes. Dehydration also may impair performance in prolonged intermittent, high-intensity anaerobic sports such as soccer and tennis.

Fluid supplementation is theorized to prevent fatigue associated with dehydration during prolonged exercise under warm environmental conditions by helping prevent impairment of cardiovascular functions or temperature regulation.

Effectiveness

Thousands of research studies have been conducted to investigate the effect of dehydration and fluid-replenishment techniques on body temperature regulation and physical performance. Two techniques have been found to help prevent the adverse effects of dehydration on aerobic endurance exercise in warm or hot environments. Rehydration involves the consumption of fluid supplements during the exercise bout itself, whereas hyperhydration involves the intake of fluids prior to exercise. Of the two, rehydration is the most effective means of preventing the adverse effects of dehydration during exercise. However, when compared to conditions in which no fluid is ingested, both techniques have been reported to (a) delay the onset of dehydration, (b) help maintain cardiovascular function, (c) reduce the magnitude of the rise in body temperature, and (d) improve performance during prolonged aerobic exercise in the heat (figure 8.17).

Research suggests that in sport events of less than 1 hour's duration, water supplementation alone is adequate. In events greater than 1 hour, fluids containing carbohydrate may be more effective. The additional carbohydrate will not impair the absorption or utilization of water, but may help to maintain blood glucose levels and provide a source of energy for the muscle.

Safety

Fluid supplementation is safe and actually may help prevent serious heat illnesses that can occur when exercising in the heat. Fluids containing carbohydrate and other nutrients are also safe, although highly concentrated carbohydrate solutions may cause gastrointestinal distress in some individuals.

Legal and Ethical Aspects

Fluid supplementation is legal and ethical in conjunction with sport competition.

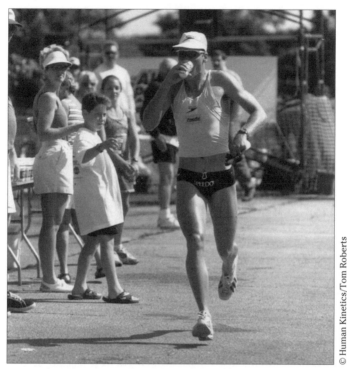

Figure 8.17 Sport drinks may be an effective means for replacing both fluids and carbohydrates during prolonged aerobic endurance events.

Recommendations

If you plan to exercise or compete under warm environmental conditions, both rehydration and hyperhydration techniques are highly recommended. Fluid replacement recommendations offered by the American College of Sports Medicine (ACSM) or other investigators may serve as a useful guide.

1. To hyperhydrate, consume adequate amounts of fluids in the 24 hours prior to exercise. Consume 500 milliliters (about 17 ounces) of cold fluid within 2 hours before exercise. Additional water may be consumed intermittently up to the start of exercise.

2. To rehydrate during exercise, drink fluids early and try to replace body fluids lost through sweating. Sweat rates vary among athletes, so you might want to determine your sweat losses as suggested in the sidebar. For example, if you calculate that you lose about 2 pounds, or 1 quart, of body water during exercise, then you should attempt to consume that much fluid, or as much as you can tolerate, during

exercise. Drinking 8 ounces (about 240 milliliters) of fluid every 15 minutes would be adequate in this case.

A good way to determine your body water losses is to weigh yourself nude both before and after your typical exercise bout. Also, measure accurately the amount of fluid you have consumed during exercise. If you exercise for 1 hour, consume 1 pint (about 470 milliliters, or 1 pound) of fluid, and weigh 1 pound less afterwards, you lost about 2 pounds or about 1 quart (about .95 liter) of sweat during the exercise bout.

3. If you are exercising for more than 1 hour and want to include carbohydrate in your fluid supplement, the general recommendation is to consume about 30 to 60 grams of carbohydrate per hour. Consumption of 1 liter, a little over a quart, of a 6 percent carbohydrate sport drink will provide 60 grams of carbohydrate. Table 8.9 indicates the amount of fluid you would have to consume to obtain 30–60 grams of carbohydrate from sport drinks with a 6 percent to 10 percent carbohydrate concentration.

4. Rehydrate after exercise. Thirst usually is a good guide for helping replace fluid losses over the next 24 hours. Also, consume foods with adequate amounts of salt to replace the sodium and chloride losses in sweat.

Folic Acid

Classification and Usage

Folic acid, an essential B vitamin, may be classified as a nutritional sports ergogenic. Folic acid is a water-soluble vitamin found in natural foods such as liver, whole-grain products, dry beans, dark green leafy vegetables, and fruits. The Recommended Dietary Allowance (RDA) for folic acid is 200 micrograms per day for adults. Some nutritionists recommend higher levels, 400 micrograms per day, for females of childbearing age because folic acid may help prevent birth defects.

Folic acid supplements are available individually or as part of a multivitamin/multimineral complex. Some sport drinks are fortified with folic acid. Studies investigating the ergogenic effect of folic acid supplementation have used dosages of up to 5 milligrams per day for several months.

Sports Performance Factor

Physical power. Folic acid supplementation has been studied in attempts to increase aerobic power and endurance for sport events that derive energy from the oxygen energy systems.

Theory

Folic acid functions as a coenzyme involved in the synthesis of DNA, the genetic material within the cell nucleus. Because DNA is needed to regenerate red blood cells (RBCs) in the bone marrow, folic acid supplementation has been theorized to facilitate the replacement of RBCs damaged during training.

Effectiveness

Although a folic acid deficiency could impair aerobic endurance performance, no scientific data are available to indicate that folic acid supplementation is an effective sports ergogenic for well-nourished athletes. For example, although folate supplementation did improve the serum folate status in female, folate-deficient marathon runners, it did not improve (a) VO_2max, (b) maximal treadmill running time, (c) peak lactate levels, or (d) running speed at the anaerobic (lactate) threshold.

Safety

Folic acid is considered a safe vitamin supplement even in megadoses hundreds of times the RDA, although there are no reasons to ingest such amounts. Excess folic acid might prevent detection of a vitamin B_{12} deficiency.

Legal and Ethical Aspects

Folic acid supplementation is legal and ethical in conjunction with sport competition.

Recommendations

Based on the available scientific evidence, folic acid supplementation is not an effective sports ergogenic, and its use is not recommended.

Ideally, most athletes should obtain adequate folic acid through their diets by consuming a variety of wholesome, natural foods. A basic once-a-day vitamin tablet with supplemental folic acid of up to 400 micrograms may benefit some athletes, including (a) those in weight-control sports on very-low-calorie diets, and (b) female athletes of childbearing age to help prevent birth defects.

Ginseng

Classification and Usage

Ginseng is a dietary supplement that may be classified as a nutritional sports ergogenic. Ginseng is the general term for a variety of natural chemical extracts derived from the plant family Araliaceae. Ginseng extracts contain chemicals that may influence human physiology, the most important being the glycosides, or ginsenosides. Ginseng extracts, and their physiologic effects, vary depending on the plant species, the part of the plant used, and the place of origin.

The most common forms of ginseng include Chinese or Korean (Panax ginseng), American (Panax quinquefolium), Japanese (Panax japonicum), and Russian/Siberian (Eleutherococcus senticosus). Eleutherococcus senticosus is recognized as a legitimate form of ginseng and its ginsenosides also are referred to as eleutherosides.

Commercial ginseng preparations are sold in capsule and liquid form. Many different types containing ginsenosides or eleutherosides are found in health food stores, drug stores, and even supermarkets (figure 8.18). Recommended dosages vary depending on the type and form of the ginseng product. Dosages used in research have varied, but normally coincided with the recommendations of the ginseng product manufacturer. Commercial products may suffer from lack of quality control. A recent assay of 50 commercial ginseng preparations indicated 44 contained ginsenoside concentrations ranging from 1.9 to 9.0 percent and six of the products contained no detectable ginsenosides. One product contained large amounts of ephedrine, a stimulant prohibited by the International Olympic Committee.

Sports Performance Factor

Physical power. Ginseng supplementation has been studied in attempts to increase physical power from all three human energy systems, the ATP-CP, lactic acid, and oxygen energy systems.

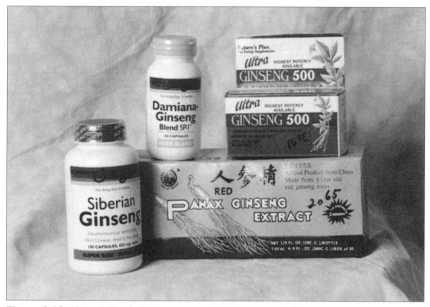

Figure 8.18 A variety of ginseng preparations are available.

Theory

The most prevalent theory suggests that ginseng may activate the hypothalamic-pituitary-adrenal cortex axis. In brief, ginseng is believed to stimulate the hypothalamus in the brain. The hypothalamus controls the pituitary gland, the master endocrine gland that secretes hormones controlling other endocrine glands in the body, including the adrenal gland. The adrenal cortex secretes cortisol, a hormone involved in the response to stress. Russian researchers used the term *adaptogens* to depict the physiologic activity of ginseng. One of the major actions of an adaptogen is an increased resistance to the catabolic effects of stress, including physical stress such as strenuous exercise, possibly by exerting favorable effects on the secretion of cortisol.

Several related theories suggest ginseng supplementation may enhance muscle glycogen synthesis after exercise, may help sustain muscle creatine phosphate (CP) during strenuous exercise, decrease lactic acid levels during exercise, and exert a positive effect on nitrogen or protein balance. In essence, given these theorized antistress effects, ginseng supplementation is theorized to enhance sports performance by allowing athletes to train more intensely or to induce an antifatiguing effect and increase stamina during competition. Such an effect could benefit most athletes.

Other theories have been proposed to explain the potential ergogenic effect on aerobic endurance capacity, again partly through the effect of ginseng on the hypothalamus. The hypothalamus also exerts control over the sympathetic nervous system, the part of the central nervous system that controls numerous autonomic functions, including the heart and blood vessels. Theoretically, hypothalamic stimulation could improve cardiac function and increase blood flow during exercise. Related theories suggest ginseng supplementation may increase hemoglobin levels, increase oxygen extraction by the muscle, and improve mitochondria metabolism in the muscle. Collectively, these theories suggest an enhanced oxygen delivery to and utilization in the muscle, the two key factors in the oxygen energy system.

Although numerous theories have been advanced in attempts to explain the alleged ergogenic effects of ginseng supplementation, an underlying mechanism has yet to be determined.

Effectiveness

Many of the advertised claims of increased energy and performance associated with ginseng supplementation are based on studies conducted in the 1960s and 1970s. Although numerous studies investigated the ergogenic possibilities of ginseng supplementation, few were well controlled. Research design flaws included no control or placebo group, no double-blind protocol, no randomization of order of treatment, and no statistical analysis.

Russian researchers were particularly interested in Russian/Siberian ginseng, or Eleutherococcus senticosus (ES), and generally reported favorable effects of ES supplementation on various measures of physical performance. Analysis of the Russian research is difficult, however, because the actual dosages and methodology generally are not fully described. Through personal correspondence, an emigrant Russian physician who worked with Soviet athletes confided that Russian scientists were pressured to produce positive results with their ES research. Many studies were not blinded, so Soviet athletes who believed that ES was an effective nutritional ergogenic may have benefited from the placebo effect. The Russian research findings appear to be unreliable; one reviewer noted recently that there were methodological problems with all of the Russian studies.

Other than the Russian studies with ES, most other studies during the 1960s and 1970s investigated the ergogenic effect of other forms of ginseng, usually commercial preparations. Many of these studies also suffered from lack of appropriate experimental design and some were funded by the manufacturer or distributor of the commercial product studied. One study was well designed, but the commercial preparation contained additional ingredients that might exert ergogenic effects. Highlighting these methodological problems in a recent extensive review of the ergogenic effect of ginseng supplementation, Michael Bahrke and William Morgan concluded that there is a lack of controlled research demonstrating the ability of ginseng to improve or prolong performance.

Subsequent to the review by Bahrke and Morgan, four well-controlled studies evaluated the ergogenic effects of standardized ginseng extracts, including commercial products containing Eleutherococcus senticosus, and reported no significant effects on various performance measures, including metabolic (oxygen uptake and lactic acid accumulation) and physiological (heart rate and ventilation) responses to submaximal and maximal running, psychological ratings of perceived exertion, mood states, or cycling and running time to exhaustion.

Currently, well-controlled research does not support the effectiveness of ginseng supplementation as a sports ergogenic.

Safety

Commercial ginseng preparations appear to have relatively low acute or chronic toxicity when taken in dosages recommended by the manufacturer. However, a ginseng-abuse syndrome has been reported, with such symptoms as high blood pressure, nervousness, and sleeplessness. These effects may be attributed to the postulated stimulant effect of ginseng, or possibly to additional substances in the commercial preparation, such as the stimulant ephedrine. (See Ephedrine.)

Legal and Ethical Aspects

Ginseng supplementation as a sports ergogenic is both legal and ethical, unless commercial ginseng products contain prohibited substances, such as ephedrine.

Recommendations

Ginseng supplementation is not recommended as a sports ergogenic because no reputable scientific data support its effectiveness to enhance performance.

However, ginseng has survived as a tonic for thousands of years, suggesting there may be some associated benefits. Most studies investigating the ergogenic potential of ginseng supplementation used short-term periods of supplementation, usually 6 to 8 weeks or less. Some research suggests long-term ginseng supplementation may prevent some adverse effects of stress on the immune system. Although not studied extensively in athletes, a healthier immune system could help prevent illness or some of the symptoms of the overtraining syndrome during high-intensity training. Individuals who wish to experiment with long-term ginseng supplementation should consult with their physicians, because ginseng use may exacerbate various health problems, such as high blood pressure. Long-term use may lead to the ginseng-abuse syndrome.

Glycerol

Classification and Usage

Glycerol may be classified as a physiological sports ergogenic. It is a sweet, colorless, liquid alcohol found naturally in fats that we eat. Glycerol is produced commercially from hydrolysis of fats for use in food products, cough medicines, and skin-care products. Drugstores may carry glycerol labeled as glycerin or glycerine in the skin-care section; glycerol is also available as Glycerate in packet form. A sports drink containing glycerol has also been advertised recently.

Dosages used in research are based on body weight or total body water, and have approximated 1 gram of glycerin per kilogram body weight with each gram diluted in about 20 to 25 milliliters of water or similar fluid.

Sports Performance Factor

Physical power. Glycerol supplementation has been studied in attempts to enhance aerobic power and endurance performance, particularly under warm environmental conditions.

Theory

Glycerol is theorized to prevent fatigue associated with dehydration during prolonged exercise under warm environmental conditions, but may enhance performance by other mechanisms as well, such as by an increased blood volume.

Dehydration may impair performance in prolonged aerobic endurance events. To help deter dehydration, athletes consume fluids to

> **A**necdote: At the 1991 World Championships in Tokyo, held in hot, humid conditions, the four U. S. marathoners who used glycerol finished their races, while two others who didn't take glycerol dropped out.
> —*Amby Burfoot, executive editor,* Runner's World

hyperhydrate before and rehydrate during the event. Glycerol supplementation is theorized to enhance the hyperhydration effect, helping the body store more water compared to hyperhydration with water alone. It also may be consumed in a rehydration fluid during exercise.

Effectiveness

Some research supports the theory that glycerol supplementation in fluids, compared to water hyperhydration alone, increases total body water stores, including the plasma volume in the blood. Research findings are not extensive and the findings are equivocal. Several studies indicate that glycerol-induced hyperhydration may help maintain a lower heart rate and body core temperature during exercise under heat stress conditions, and may enhance prolonged aerobic endurance capacity in cyclists riding to exhaustion. Conversely, other studies indicate glycerol-induced hyperhydration exerted no effect on temperature regulation, physiological responses during exercise, or prolonged cycling tasks of approximately 3 hours.

Safety

Labels on glycerin products indicate not to use the product internally, but when diluted with fluids as noted above, glycerol supplementation appears to be safe. However, glycerol may cause headaches and nausea; patients who are pregnant or who have high blood pressure, diabetes, or kidney problems should consult with their physician before trying glycerol supplementation.

Legal and Ethical Aspects

The IOC prohibits intravenous infusion of glycerol, but oral solutions are legal. Although fats contain glycerol in a glyceride form, pure glycerol is not a normal dietary constituent. Thus, glycerol supplementation may contravene the general meaning of the International Olympic Committee anti-doping legislation, i.e., consuming a substance in abnormal quantities with the intent of artificially and unfairly enhancing sports performance. Depending on the viewpoint of the athlete, glycerol supplementation may be either ethical or unethical.

Recommendations

Some research, although limited, provides support for the theory, effectiveness, and safety of glycerol supplementation, at least in accordance with amounts recommended above. Exceeding the recommended amount may be dangerous. Glycerol supplementation has enhanced performance in prolonged cycling in one study, but not in another. Additional well-controlled research is needed to evaluate the ergogenic potential of glycerol-induced hyperhydration. Research is also needed to see the effect on running performance because carrying extra water weight may decrease running efficiency. Given the general overtone of the IOC anti-doping legislation, the use of glycerol supplementation may be considered unethical.

For those who wish to experiment with glycerol hyperhydration, one procedure is presented in table 8.12.

TABLE 8.12
One Procedure for Glycerol Hyperhydration

1. Determine your body weight in kilograms (multiply your weight in pounds by .454).

2. Consume one gram of glycerol per kilogram body weight. If you weigh 70 kilograms (154 pounds), you would consume 70 grams of glycerol.

3. Glycerol, as glycerin or Glycerate, should not be consumed full-strength, but must be diluted in other fluids before drinking.

4. With Glycerate or similar commercial products, follow the instructions on the packet. With glycerine, make a 5 percent solution with water. Add 50 grams of glycerin to a liter (1,000 milliliters) of water, or about 1.5 ounces of glycerin in a quart of water. Each 100 milliliters of fluid contains 5 grams of glycerol, so to obtain 70 grams, our 70-kilogram athlete must drink about 1,400 milliliters of the glycerin-water mixture (100 milliliters/5 x 70 kilograms = 1,400 milliliters).

5. Consume the fluid from 2.5 to 1.5 hours before exercise.

HMB (Beta-hydroxy-beta-methylbutyrate)

Classification and Usage

Beta-hydroxy-beta-methylbutyrate (HMB) may be classified as a nutritional sports ergogenic. HMB is a byproduct of leucine metabolism in the human body. Leucine, a natural amino acid constituent of dietary protein, is the normal source of HMB production in the body, which averages about .2 to .4 gram per day depending on dietary leucine intake. HMB is marketed as a dietary supplement and is available commercially as calcium-HMB-monohydrate. Typical doses used in research approximated a total of 1.5–3.0 grams per day taken in multiple doses; some scientists recommend the total dose be consumed in three or four equal amounts throughout the day. HMB is a patented product, so check for the patent number by Metabolic Technologies, Incorporated (MTI) because some fake HMB products are also being marketed, e.g., histidine, methionine, and B vitamins.

Sports Performance Factor

Mechanical edge and physical power. HMB has been studied primarily in attempts to increase muscle mass and decrease body fat for enhanced strength and power or for a more aesthetic physical appearance in sports such as bodybuilding.

Theory

Investigators do not know how HMB supplementation may help to increase lean muscle mass or decrease body fat, but they offer several hypotheses. Through some unknown mechanism, possibly by being incorporated into cell components or influencing cellular enzyme activity, HMB may inhibit the breakdown of muscle tissue during strenuous exercise; this prevailing hypothesis is supported by urine and blood tests showing fewer metabolic byproducts of exercise-induced muscle damage following HMB supplementation.

Effectiveness

Several animal studies involving poultry, cattle, and pigs have indicated HMB supplementation may increase lean muscle mass and decrease body fat. Although scientific data involving humans is less extensive, three preliminary studies from Iowa State University have revealed some supportive findings.

In the first study, which appears to be the best controlled of the three, HMB supplementation significantly increased lean tissue and strength in untrained males who initiated a resistance-training program for 3 weeks. The subjects consumed either 0, 1.5 grams, or 3.0 grams of HMB per day, and although all subjects increased lean tissue mass and strength with the resistance training programs, the HMB groups gained significantly more, generally in linear relationship to the dose. That is to say, the group taking 3.0 grams HMB gained more than those taking 1.5 grams per day.

In the second study, which was not controlled as well, HMB supplementation (3.0 grams per day) did not increase total body mass, decrease body fat, or improve performance in two of three strength tests in physically active males who continued resistance training several hours per day over a 50-day period. Body composition was determined seven times over the duration of the study and, compared to the placebo group, HMB supplementation did increase lean muscle mass during several of the intermediate test periods, but not at the completion of the study. Additionally, although participants in the HMB group significantly increased strength in the 1-repetition maximal bench press, they did not increase strength in the squat or hang clean tests.

In the third study, with few details available, HMB supplementation (3.0 grams per day) increased lean body mass, decreased fat mass, and increased bench press strength in both trained and untrained subjects over a 4-week period of resistance training. HMB supplementation increased bench press strength 55 percent more than did the placebo group. The investigators conducted other strength tests and although gains seemed to be higher in the HMB group, there were no significant differences compared to the placebo group.

These preliminary findings are intriguing, but several caveats are in order. First, these studies were conducted by the same laboratory group that developed HMB. Although this is a well-respected research laboratory, corroborating data from other laboratories are needed to confirm these preliminary findings. Second, the techniques used to measure strength varied between the studies, and the technique used in the first study is not commonly accepted as a standardized strength-testing procedure. Third, the placebo used in one study was likely not a true placebo because it appeared to vary in appearance compared to the HMB treatment. Fourth, although most studies used multiple tests of strength, improvements were noted only in some, not all, of the tests.

These caveats do not detract from the importance of these studies, but they do suggest the information currently available regarding the ergogenic effectiveness of HMB supplementation is preliminary, and more scientific data are needed before HMB can be confirmed as a useful sports ergogenic.

Safety

HMB supplementation appears to be safe. No adverse effects of chronic supplementation have been noted in animals. In human studies, there have been no reported adverse acute side effects from HMB supplementation up to 4.0 grams per day for several weeks. Although HMB supplementation may increase serum HMB levels, serum values of other constituents remain unchanged.

Legal and Ethical Aspects

HMB supplementation is legal. Currently there does not appear to be an ethical problem with its use in conjunction with sports performance.

Recommendations

Although the effectiveness of HMB supplementation as an effective sports ergogenic remains to be proven, the preliminary data are somewhat supportive and it appears to be a safe, legal, and ethical supplement. Athletes involved in resistance training might experiment with it, taking careful measurements of body mass, body segments, and strength while supplementing. Endurance athletes who train intensely might benefit if HMB would prevent muscle tissue degradation, but we have little information relative to the effect of HMB supplementation on aerobic endurance athletes. One consideration may be the expense because HMB supplements are rather costly.

Human Growth Hormone (hGH)

Classification and Usage

Human growth hormone (hGH) may be classified as a physiologic sports ergogenic. A natural hormone, hGH is secreted by the anterior pituitary gland in the brain. hGH stimulates growth of the bones, but also affects the metabolism of carbohydrate, fat, and protein. hGH is considered an anabolic hormone.

Previously, the only source of hGH was human cadavers, but through genetic engineering a synthetic form (rhGH) has been developed using recombinant technology. Technically, rhGH may be classified as a drug, or a pharmacological sports ergogenic. Since the synthetic form's appearance in 1985, several surveys indicate increased rhGH use by athletes, some as young as 14 to 15 years old. Dosages utilized in research with young males approximated 40 micrograms per kilogram body weight daily for 6 weeks. rhGH is administered by injection.

Sports Performance Factor

Mechanical edge and physical power. rhGH is used primarily to increase muscle mass and decrease body fat for enhanced strength and power or for a more aesthetic physical appearance in sports such as bodybuilding. Prepubertal and adolescent athletes may use hGH to maximize height.

Theory

Supplemental rhGH is designed to increase the total hGH supply in the body, which may stimulate the production of another hormone, insulin-like growth factor-1, that spurs growth of muscle tissue. Increased hGH may accelerate the oxidation of fat.

Effectiveness

When administered to subjects who are hGH-deficient, rhGH supplementation increases lean body mass and decreases body fat. When given to subjects who have normal endogenous levels of hGH, rhGH supplementation may increase lean body mass, but not necessarily muscle mass, strength, or athletic performance. Several studies have investigated the effect of rhGH supplementation on body composition and strength in young males with normal rhGH levels undergoing strenuous resistance training. In general, rhGH supplementation did increase lean body mass. However, magnetic resonance imaging (MRI) techniques indicated that the increased overall lean body mass was not contractile muscle tissue, but possibly increased size of other tissues (such as the spleen), or water retention. Moreover, there was no improvement in strength attributable to rhGH supplementation. Several well-controlled studies have reported comparable findings with rhGH supplementation to experienced resistance-trained athletes.

Safety

Although no data are available detailing adverse health effects in athletes, excess secretion of hGH by the anterior pituitary in adults is associated with acromegaly, or thickening of soft tissues in the face, hands, and feet. Excess hGH may also cause pathological enlargement of body organs, such as the liver, kidneys, and heart, which may predispose athletes to chronic diseases such as diabetes and cardiac myopathy. rhGH must be injected, increasing the risk of various infections, such as hepatitis and AIDS, from contaminated needles. Thus, use of rhGH may pose some significant health risks and such risks may become evident in the future if athletes increase and sustain the use of rhGH.

Legal and Ethical Aspects

rhGH supplementation is prohibited by most athletic governing bodies and is considered unethical behavior. rhGH use is not detectable using current drug-testing procedures, but the IOC has initiated a research project entitled GH2000, ostensibly to develop and implement a validated rhGH test for the 2000 Olympic Games in Sydney, Australia.

> In the year 2000 or 2004, testing for human growth hormone will be in place, but a blood test will be needed.
> —*Gary Wadler, MD, authority on drug testing*

Recommendations

Although rhGH may increase lean body mass in rhGH-normal subjects, there is no evidence of increased contractile muscle protein, strength, or athletic performance. Additionally, rhGH supplementation may also pose significant health risks and its use is illegal and unethical. For some athletes, rhGH supplementation may impair performance due to excess water retention or insulin resistance. Accordingly, rhGH supplementation is not recommended.

Inosine

Classification and Usage

Inosine is a dietary supplement that may be classified as a physiological sports ergogenic. Inosine is sold separately or in combination with other purported nutritional sports ergogenics. Usual dosages are 5 to 6 grams per day.

Sports Performance Factor

Physical power. Inosine has been studied primarily in attempts to increase aerobic power and endurance for events associated with the oxygen energy system, but has been advertised to enhance explosive power associated with the ATP-CP energy system.

Theory

Inosine is a nucleoside, an essential compound in the body with several roles in energy metabolism, some that may be potentially ergogenic. On the basis of animal research and blood storage techniques, sports nutrition entrepreneurs have advertised inosine supplementation as a means to enhance ATP production in the muscle, improve respiration, increase the ability to deliver oxygen to the muscles, metabolize blood sugars, reduce lactic acid, and improve aerobic capacity. Many of these effects have been attributed to the purported ability of inosine supplementation to increase 2,3-DPG formation (2,3-DPG is a compound in the red blood cells that facilitates the release of oxygen to the cells). Theoretically, the enhanced short-term ATP production could benefit strength athletes, whereas the other effects could enhance aerobic endurance exercise performance.

Effectiveness

Several studies have evaluated the effect of inosine supplementation with the primary focus on aerobic endurance capacity, but with some implications for anaerobic performance. The studies were well designed, using highly trained athletes in a double-blind, placebo, crossover experimental protocol. Inosine dosages ranged from 5 to 6 grams per day for 2 to 5 days. Summarizing the results of these studies, compared to the placebo trial, inosine supplementation had no ergogenic effect on: (a) 2,3-DPG; (b) lung ventilation, heart rate, or oxygen metabolism during submaximal and maximal exercise; (c) blood glucose or lactic acid levels; (d) $\dot{V}O_2$peak; (e) peak power and total work output on a cycle ergometer; or (f) 3-mile run time. Interestingly, inosine supplementation significantly impaired performance in two studies, decreasing exercise time to fatigue in both a progressive treadmill run and a constant load supramaximal cycling sprint. One study group speculated inosine supplementation may actually interfere with optimal energy production from the lactic acid energy system, which could come into play during the final stages of an aerobic endurance task, such as a prolonged sprint to the finish line.

Safety

Inosine appears to be a safe dietary supplement in the doses advertised, but one study did report a significant increase in uric acid. Uric acid is the end byproduct of inosine catabolism and may elicit symptoms of gouty arthritis, particularly pain in the knee and foot joints.

Legal and Ethical Aspects

Inosine supplementation is legal and ethical.

Recommendations

Inosine supplementation is not recommended as a means of improving sports performance. There are no scientific data supporting a sports ergogenic effect; inosine supplementation may impair performance in some events and may increase the risk for gouty arthritis.

Iron

Classification and Usage

Iron, an essential mineral, may be classified as a nutritional sports ergogenic. Dietary iron comes in two forms. Animal foods such as meat, fish, and poultry contain heme iron, while nonheme iron is found primarily in plant foods such as whole-grain products, dark-green leafy vegetables, and dried fruits. The Recommended Dietary Allowance is 10 milligrams for adult males, 12 milligrams for teenage males, and 15 milligrams for teenage and adult females.

Iron supplements are available as iron salts, such as iron fumarate and iron sulfate. Dosages used in research have varied depending on the iron status of the subject.

Sports Performance Factor

Physical power. Iron supplements are used in attempts to increase aerobic power and endurance for sport events that derive energy primarily from the oxygen energy system.

Theory

Iron is a component of hemoglobin in the red blood cell (RBC), myoglobin in the muscle cell, and some of the oxidative enzymes within the mitochondria (see figure 8.19). Hemoglobin and myoglobin are carriers of oxygen, while the iron-based oxidative enzymes are

During the Tour of Italy, the great American cyclist Greg LeMond was doing poorly. His trainer suggested LeMond was suffering from iron deficiency. After several days of iron injections he began to improve, winning the final time trial. He continued to improve, and went on to win the Tour de France about a month later.

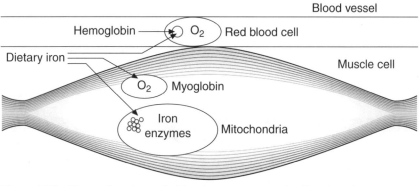

Figure 8.19 Dietary iron is needed for the transport and utilization of oxygen.

essential in the formation of ATP in the oxygen energy system. Theoretically, iron supplementation is designed to maximize the function of the oxygen energy system and improve performance in aerobic endurance exercise tasks.

Effectiveness

Epidemiological research conducted relative to the iron status of athletes has revealed three conditions. Most male and female athletes have normal hemoglobin levels and normal body iron stores. Some male endurance athletes, some female athletes, and many female endurance athletes have normal hemoglobin levels but low body iron stores—a condition known as iron deficiency without anemia. A small number of female athletes, particularly distance runners, have both subnormal hemoglobin levels and subnormal body iron stores—a condition known as iron-deficiency anemia.

Iron supplements have been used to improve performance in all three conditions. As might be expected, the remediation of iron-deficiency anemia with the return to normal hemoglobin levels through iron supplementation helped to return exercise performance to normal. On the other hand, iron supplementation to athletes with normal hemoglobin levels and iron status had no influence upon endurance performance.

The results of research with subjects who have iron deficiency without anemia are contradictory. Most studies show that iron supplementation will improve iron status, but not $\dot{V}O_2$max and exercise performance. However, a few studies have noted that the return of normal iron status in nonanemic female athletes following iron supplementation was associated with improved markers of enhanced oxidative metabolism in the muscle during exercise and improved running performance. Nevertheless, a recent review of the relevant research concluded that iron supplementation to athletes who were iron-deficient but nonanemic would not improve physical performance.

In summary, iron supplementation does not appear to enhance exercise performance unless an iron-deficiency anemia is cured. However, it is possible that some individual iron-deficient, nonanemic athletes may benefit if oxidative functions in the muscle are improved.

Safety

Iron supplementation in amounts no larger than the RDA appear to be safe. Black stools are common, and either constipation or diarrhea may occur. About two to three people out of 1,000 are predisposed to hemochromatosis. Hemochromatosis is caused by excessive storage of iron in the body, particularly in the liver, which may lead to cirrhosis and possible death.

Legal and Ethical Aspects

Iron supplements are legal and ethical.

Recommendations

In general, iron supplementation is not recommended as a sports ergogenic for athletes with normal hemoglobin and iron status because it has not been found to effectively enhance sports performance.

Athletes concerned about their hemoglobin or iron status should have an appropriate blood test by sports-oriented health professionals. If an iron deficiency is evident, appropriate iron therapy may be prescribed. Additionally, athletes who may be "going to altitude" to train may need an iron prescription. Altitude training stimulates the formation of new RBCs, which need more iron for the formation of hemoglobin.

Ideally, most athletes should obtain adequate iron through their diets, selecting foods rich in heme and nonheme iron as noted in table 8.13. Heme iron, found in meat, is better absorbed into the body than nonheme iron, but vitamin C facilitates the absorption of nonheme iron. Drink orange juice with your toast in the morning.

If foods are not selected wisely, a basic one-per-day mineral tablet may benefit some athletes, including (a) those who abstain from meat products, (b) those who participate in weight-control sports, and (c) female endurance athletes. In such cases, the recommended procedure is to supplement the normal dietary iron intake with about 10 to

> **TABLE 8.13**
> Iron Content of Common Foods in the Food Exchanges
> and Fast Foods

Milk
1 cup 1% fat milk = .1 milligram
1 cup nonfat yogurt = .2 milligram

Meat/fish/poultry/cheese
1 ounce Swiss cheese = .05 milligram
1 ounce lean steak = 1 milligram
1 ounce shrimp = .3 milligram

Breads/cereals/legumes/starchy vegetables
1 slice whole-wheat bread = .85 milligram
1 cup baked beans = .7 milligram
1 cup corn = 1.4 milligrams

Vegetables
1 cup cooked broccoli = 1.3 milligrams
1 cup cooked spinach = 6.4 milligrams

Fruits
1 banana = .3 milligram
1/4 cup raisins = .8 milligram

Fast foods
1 Burger King BK broiler = 3.2 milligrams
1 Wendy's quarter pound hamburger = 4.7 milligrams

15 milligrams, the normal amount found in the typical once-a-day vitamin/mineral supplement. Some breakfast cereals are fortified with 10 to 15 milligrams of iron per serving which may substitute for the pill form. Do not take iron supplements greater than the RDA indiscriminately.

Magnesium

Classification and Usage

Magnesium, an essential mineral, may be classified as a nutritional sports ergogenic. Magnesium is a natural constituent of various foods, particularly nuts, seafood, whole-grain products, dark-green leafy vegetables, and fruits and vegetables. The Recommended Dietary Allowance is 350 milligrams for males and 280 milligrams for females.

Magnesium supplements are available in a variety of forms, including magnesium citrate and magnesium carbonate. In some studies, magnesium supplements of 200–300 milligrams have been used to double the normal daily intake.

Sports Performance Factor

Mechanical edge and physical power. Magnesium supplements have been studied in attempts to increase physical power in the ATP-CP energy system, primarily by increasing muscle mass. Additionally, magnesium supplements have been studied in attempts to increase aerobic power and endurance for events dependent on the oxygen energy system.

Theory

Magnesium plays a role in more than 300 enzymatic reactions in the human body, many involving carbohydrate, fat, and protein metabolism. Magnesium supplementation is theorized to enhance protein synthesis, particularly muscle mass with implications for increased strength and power. Magnesium supplementation is also theorized to enhance carbohydrate and fatty acid metabolism, which could benefit aerobic endurance capacity.

Effectiveness

In general, there are no studies available indicating that magnesium supplementation will increase sports performance in trained individuals with adequate magnesium status. One study did report an increased strength in untrained subjects following 7 weeks of magnesium supplementation and resistance training, but no strength improvements were noted in trained marathon runners following 10 weeks of magnesium supplementation.

Two studies have reported that magnesium supplementation improved the energy efficiency for running and rowing, as evidenced by either a lower oxygen cost or less lactic acid production, but no effect on performance was noted. Other studies have not shown any favorable effect of magnesium supplementation on aerobic performance, including marathon running performance.

One reviewer has noted that magnesium status has not been determined in some of these studies. One of the symptoms of magnesium deficiency is muscular weakness, so if magnesium supplementation corrects a deficiency, muscular performance could be enhanced.

Safety

Magnesium supplementation in amounts no larger than the RDA appear to be safe. Excessive magnesium intake may cause nausea, vomiting, and diarrhea, and may interfere with the absorption of calcium and other minerals.

Legal and Ethical Aspects

Magnesium supplementation is legal and ethical.

TABLE 8.14
Magnesium Content of Common Foods in the Food Exchanges

Milk
  1 cup 1% fat milk = 34 milligrams
  1 cup nonfat yogurt = 43 milligrams

Meat/fish/poultry/cheese
  1 ounce Swiss cheese = 10 milligrams
  1 ounce lean steak = 9 milligrams
  1 ounce shrimp = 10 milligrams

Breads/cereals/legumes/starchy vegetables
  1 slice whole-wheat bread = 23 milligrams
  1 cup baked beans = 81 milligrams
  1 cup corn = 30 milligrams

Vegetables
  1 cup cooked broccoli = 37 milligrams
  1 cup cooked spinach = 157 milligrams

Fruits
  1 banana = 33 milligrams
  1/4 cup raisins = 12 milligrams

Fast foods
  1 Burger King BK broiler = 29 milligrams
  1 Wendy's quarter-pound hamburger = 49 milligrams

Recommendations

In general, magnesium supplementation is not recommended as a sports ergogenic because it has not been found to effectively enhance sport performance.

Ideally, athletes should obtain adequate magnesium through their diets, selecting foods rich in magnesium as noted in table 8.14. If foods are not selected wisely, however, athletes who participate in weight-control sports might benefit from a magnesium supplement containing the RDA of 280–350 milligrams.

Marijuana

Classification and Usage

Marijuana may be classified as a pharmacological sports ergogenic. Marijuana is composed of the shredded, dried leaves, flowers, and stems of the cannabis sativa plant (figure 8.20) that contain the psychoactive substance, delta-9-tetrahydrocannabinol (THC). Marijuana typically is smoked, but may be consumed orally. A typical 1.5-gram marijuana cigarette with 1.5 percent THC contains approximately 21 milligrams THC, enough for a pharmacological effect. Physical performance has been studied from 10 minutes to 24 hours after smoking marijuana.

Sports Performance Factor

Mental strength. Marijuana has been studied in attempts to enhance various sports performance factors that may be influenced by either a supplemental stimulant or depressant effect.

Theory

Marijuana is believed to influence the function of several neurotransmitters in the brain. Depending on the interaction of these neurotransmitters, the resultant effects may be characteristic of psychological arousal or psychological relaxation.

Psychological arousal might be reflective of a sympathomimetic effect that may be associated with several physiological, and possibly ergogenic, responses, including dilation of the respiratory passageways and increased blood flow to the muscle.

Psychological relaxation may enhance precision sports performance by reducing the adverse effects of anxiety on motor control.

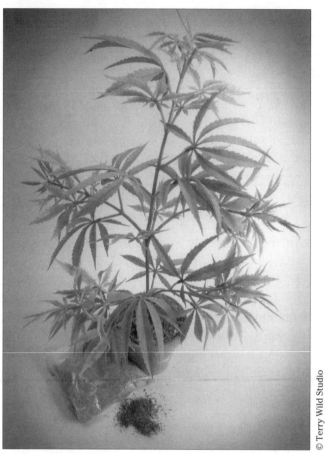

© Terry Wild Studio

Figure 8.20 Marijuana leaves represent the source of the psychoactive ingredient, delta-9-tetrahydrocannabinol.

Effectiveness

No research is available indicating that marijuana use enhances any sports performance factor. Actually, research indicates that heavy marijuana smoking may impair complex perceptual-motor performance just after smoking and even 24 hours later. Marijuana smoking also may impair heart rate responses to exercise, which has been associated with a 6.2 percent impairment in cycling performance.

Safety

Although key investigators note that marijuana is perceived as a relatively safe social drug, they also note that the state of knowledge is too limited to rule out the possibility of adverse health effects; some have been reported, including respiratory problems associated with smoking, impairment of cell-mediated immune responses, depressed reproductive functions, and development of female breast appearance in male athletes. Additionally, marijuana use may impair automobile driving ability.

Legal and Ethical Aspects

Marijuana use is not prohibited by the IOC or the USOC, but its use is prohibited by the national governing bodies for many sports and may be tested for at their request. A positive test may lead to sanctions. Additionally, other athletic governing bodies, such as the NCAA, may ban the use of marijuana, presumably due to its illegality. Its use in conjunction with sports performance would not be considered unethical, unless prohibited; however, marijuana use may be unethical because its possession and use is considered criminal behavior in many countries.

Recommendations

Research indicates that marijuana use may impair sports performance, not enhance it. Additionally, social use of marijuana has been associated with an amotivational syndrome, characterized by apathy and a lack of motivation, which may impair physical and mental training for sport. Furthermore, marijuana use may increase health risks and is a criminal offense. For these reasons, the ergogenic or social use of marijuana by athletes is not recommended.

Multivitamin/Mineral Supplements

Classification and Usage

Vitamin/mineral supplements may be classified as a nutritional sports ergogenic. Typical commercial one-per-day supplements contain up to 100 percent of the RDA for almost all essential vitamins and minerals. Other supplements may contain only specific vitamins or minerals, such as the eight vitamins in the B complex, the three antioxidant vitamins, or combinations of vitamins and minerals for a certain ergogenic purpose. Megadose capsules are common, often containing many times the RDA for some vitamins and minerals. Still other products contain additional dietary constituents, such as creatine or choline. Some sport drinks and sport bars are fortified with multiple vitamins and minerals.

Studies investigating the ergogenic effect of multivitamin/mineral supplementation have used dosages ranging from 10 to 50 times the Recommended Dietary Allowance for 3 to 9 months.

Sports Performance Factor

Physical power and mental strength. Multivitamin/mineral supplements may be used in attempts to increase all types of physical power from the three human energy systems, the ATP-CP, lactic acid, and oxygen energy systems. Additionally, thiamin and several other B vitamins may be used in attempts to improve mental strength by inducing a calmative effect.

Theory

Vitamins and minerals are involved in almost all metabolic processes in the human body, many important to sports performance as highlighted in table 8.15. Functioning as coenzymes or in other metabolic roles important to exercise performance, they are (a) essential for the optimal functioning of all three human energy systems, (b) needed for the formation of red blood cells to transport oxygen, (c) involved in the formation of muscle protein, (d) required for the formation of various neurotransmitters, and (e) vital to antioxidant activity. Theoretically, if multivitamin/mineral supplementation could enhance these metabolic functions, almost every type of sports performance could be improved.

Effectiveness

Four contemporary, well-controlled studies indicate that multivitamin/mineral supplementation does not enhance sports performance. In one of the most comprehensive studies, nationally ranked athletes training at the Australian Institute of Sport were matched by gender and performance and assigned to either a placebo or treatment group. Consumption of a daily multivitamin/mineral supplement (ranging from about 100 to 5,000 percent of the Recommended Dietary Allowance) for nearly 8 months had no ergogenic effect on uniform tests of strength, anaerobic power, and aerobic endurance, or on sport-specific performance tests. At the Lausanne Consensus Conference on Sport Nutrition, international sports nutrition authorities concluded that vitamin/mineral supplements are not necessary for athletes who consume a diet adequate in both quantity and quality of foods.

Some studies suggest substantial amounts of specific B vitamin supplementation may be ergogenic under certain circumstances,

TABLE 8.15
Possible Roles of Vitamins and Minerals in Sports Performance

Vitamin/ mineral	Adult RDA or ESADDI	Possible or putative role in sports performance
Beta-carotene (vitamin A)	5,000 IU	Antioxidant; prevention of muscle tissue damage
Vitamin E (alpha-tocopherol)	12–15 IU	Antioxidant; prevention of red blood cell damage; promotion of aerobic energy production
Thiamin (vitamin B_1)	1.1–1.5 mg	Energy release from carbohydrate; formation of hemoglobin; proper nervous system functioning
Riboflavin (vitamin B_2)	1.3–1.7 mg	Energy release from carbohydrate and fat
Niacin	15–19 mg	Energy release from carbohydrate, both aerobic and anaerobic; blockage of release of free fatty acids from adipose tissue
Pyridoxine (vitamin B_6)	2.0–2.2 mg	Energy release from carbohydrate; formation of proteins; formation of hemoglobin and oxidative enzymes; proper nervous system functioning
Vitamin B_{12}	2 mcg	Involved in DNA metabolism; red blood cell production
Folic acid	200 mcg	Involved in DNA metabolism; red blood cell production
Pantothenic acid	4–7 mg	Energy production from carbohydrate and fat
Ascorbic acid (vitamin C)	60 mg	Antioxidant; increased absorption of iron; formation of epinephrine (adrenaline); promotion of aerobic energy production; formation of connective tissues; enhanced function of immune system
Calcium	800–1,200 mg	Muscle contraction; glycogen breakdown
Phosphorus (phosphate salts)	800–1,200 mg	Formation of ATP and CP; release of oxygen from red blood cells; intracellular buffer
Magnesium	280–350 mg	Muscle contraction; glucose metabolism in muscle cell; protein formation
Iron	10–15 mg	Oxygen transport by red blood cells; oxygen utilization in muscle cells
Chromium	50–200 mcg	Enhanced function of insulin
Selenium	65–80 mcg	Enhanced antioxidant activity in cells
Vanadium	Not established	Enhanced function of insulin

IU = International Units; mg = milligrams; mcg = micrograms

although these results need to be confirmed by additional research. Two studies by the same investigators found that supplementation with vitamins B_1, B_6, and B_{12} might improve pistol-firing accuracy. The large doses used, 120 to 600 milligrams each, were theorized to increase the production of neurotransmitters, most likely serotonin, to induce a relaxing, anxiolytic effect. Less anxiety, such as that manifested by a hand tremor, would improve firing accuracy.

Other investigators reported that a supplement containing vitamins B_1, B_2, B_6, B_{12}, niacin, and pantothenic acid improved repeat sprint performance in young boys training under hot environmental conditions. Substantial amounts of B vitamins, which are water-soluble, may have been excreted in sweat and thus impaired performance in subjects receiving the placebo instead of the B-complex supplement.

Safety

Multivitamin\mineral supplements within the RDA appear to be safe, but chronic use of supplements containing larger doses of certain vitamins (A, D, niacin, B_6) and many minerals may pose significant health risks.

Legal and Ethical Aspects

Multivitamin/mineral supplementation is legal and ethical in conjunction with sport competition.

Recommendations

Based on the available scientific evidence, multivitamin/mineral supplementation is not an effective sports ergogenic for most athletes, and its use is not recommended.

Selecting wholesome natural foods in adequate amounts and quality will guarantee adequate vitamin and mineral nutrition for most athletes. If foods are not selected wisely, some athletes, including (a) those who participate in weight-control sports, (b) strict vegetarians with very limited diets, and (c) those who consume substantial calories primarily from highly processed foods, may benefit from a multivitamin/mineral supplement containing the RDA for most vitamins and minerals.

Narcotic Analgesics

Classification and Usage

Narcotic analgesics may be classified as a pharmacological sports ergogenic. They are prescription drugs designed to suppress pain—

the analgesic effect. Morphine and its pharmacological analogues are classified as depressants, but they may elicit a paradoxical euphoric or stimulant effect in appropriate doses. Small doses of some narcotic analgesics may be found in cold medications as cough suppressants.

Sports Performance Factor

Mental strength. Narcotic analgesics may affect the central nervous system in various ways, but they may be used primarily in attempts to enhance various sports performance factors that could be influenced by a supplemental calmative, relaxant, or depressant effect.

Theory

By suppressing pain sensations, narcotic analgesics theoretically may enable athletes to perform well above their normal pain thresholds, which could benefit performance in a variety of sport competitions. Additionally, narcotic analgesics may reduce anxiety, possibly enhancing performance in sport events in which excess anxiety could adversely affect fine motor control, such as pistol shooting and archery.

> The purpose of the drugs was to deaden the pain in Butkus's (all-pro football player) knees, making it possible for him to play.
> —*Joseph Nocera,* Sports Illustrated *writer*

Effectiveness

Sports performances that may be dependent on high pain tolerance conceivably could be enhanced by use of narcotic analgesics, but few data are available with humans. Research has shown that morphine may increase swim time to exhaustion in untrained mice that are exposed to a severe cold stress, but has no effect on swim performance once the mice are well trained.

Several studies have investigated the effect of morphine or one of its analogues on cardiovascular, respiratory, and metabolic responses to aerobic exercise in humans. In general, the results of these studies suggest narcotic analgesics may actually impair performance. In one study with highly trained athletes performing a standardized treadmill running protocol, a morphine analogue increased oxygen consumption, an indication of reduced running efficiency, which the investigators attributed to an impairment in running coordination. One of the possible side effects of narcotic analgesics is heaviness in the limbs, which may have caused the incoordination in these athletes.

Safety

The use of narcotic analgesics by athletes may be dangerous for several reasons. First, if the pain threshold is elevated the athlete may not recognize an injury, which could become more serious if the athlete continues to perform. Second, narcotic analgesics are both psychologically and physically addictive drugs with serious social and health consequences. Third, excessive use could suppress the respiratory system and be fatal.

> **B**rett Favre, a National Football League star quarter-back, developed a dependence on narcotic-analgesic painkillers, leading to seizures with possible fatal consequences.
>
> —*Peter King,* Sports Illustrated *writer*

Legal and Ethical Aspects

The use of narcotic analgesics is prohibited by most athletic governing bodies and is considered unethical behavior. Drug testing has been effective in detection of narcotic analgesic metabolites in the urine of athletes. A list of prohibited narcotic analgesics and over-the-counter medications (which are listed under stimulants because they also contain prohibited stimulants) may be found in appendix A. Illegal possession and use of narcotic analgesics may result in criminal penalties.

Recommendations

Use of narcotic analgesics as a sports ergogenic is not recommended because it is illegal, unethical, and may significantly increase health risks. Also, based on the available scientific evidence, use of narcotic analgesics does not enhance sports performance.

Effective legal, yet safer, pharmaceuticals are available to treat pain. Athletes should consult with their physicians for suitable alternatives. Over-the-counter drugs, including nonsteroidal anti-inflammatory agents such as ibuprofen, may help alleviate minor aches and pains.

However, their use may be associated with some health risks, such as gastrointestinal bleeding with prolonged use.

Niacin

Classification and Usage

Niacin, an essential B vitamin also known as nicotinic acid, may be classified as a nutritional sports ergogenic. Niacin is a water-soluble vitamin found in natural foods, particularly those with high protein content such as meat, fish, poultry, legumes, and whole grain and enriched breads and cereals. The Recommended Dietary Allowance (RDA) for niacin is based on caloric intake, but approximates 19 milligrams for males and 15 milligrams for females.

Niacin supplements are available individually or as part of a multi-vitamin/multimineral complex. Some sport drinks are fortified with niacin. Studies investigating the ergogenic effect of niacin supplementation have used dosages ranging from 50 to 3,000 milligrams per day for several weeks.

Sports Performance Factor

Physical power. Niacin supplementation has been studied in attempts to increase power endurance and aerobic power and endurance for sport events that derive energy from the lactic acid and the oxygen energy systems.

Theory

Niacin functions as a coenzyme for several energy processes in the cell, the production of energy via anaerobic glycolysis and oxidative enzyme reactions in the mitochondria. If niacin supplementation could enhance these energy-generating processes in the muscle cell, performance in either high-intensity anaerobic events or prolonged aerobic endurance events theoretically could be improved.

Additionally, niacin supplementation may increase blood flow to the skin, decreasing the sweat rate during exercise. Conservation of body fluids could enhance prolonged aerobic endurance exercise in warm environmental conditions.

Effectiveness

Although a niacin deficiency could impair sport performance, several recent reviews of the scientific literature concluded that niacin supplementation has not been shown to be an effective sports ergogenic for well-nourished athletes. For example, niacin supplementation has failed to improve performance in a 10-mile run and in a 3.5-mile cycle time trial following a 2-hour cycling task.

Niacin supplementation may impair performance. Niacin blocks the release of free fatty acids (FFA) from the adipose tissues during exercise. FFA may be a useful source of energy to help spare the use of muscle glycogen. Studies have shown that when muscle glycogen levels are low, niacin supplementation leads to premature fatigue.

Safety

Niacin supplements within the RDA appear to be safe, but use of larger doses may be associated with headaches, nausea, and flushing and itching of the skin. Chronic niacin supplementation may cause liver damage.

Legal and Ethical Aspects

Niacin supplementation is legal and ethical in conjunction with sport competition.

Recommendations

Based on the available scientific evidence, niacin supplementation is not an effective sports ergogenic, may impair sports performance, and may have adverse side effects; hence, its use is not recommended.

Niacin need increases with increased energy expenditure, common with most athletes. Selecting wholesome natural foods, such as lean meats and whole-grain or enriched breads and cereals, will guarantee adequate niacin intake for most athletes. Athletes in weight-control sports who consume very-low-calorie diets might consider taking a typical one-per-day vitamin supplement with 100 percent of the RDA for niacin.

Nicotine

Classification and Usage

Nicotine may be classified as a pharmacological sports ergogenic. Nicotine is a social drug classified as a stimulant. It is derived from the tobacco plant and may enter the human body through use of cigarettes, smokeless tobacco, nicotine gum, or nicotine patches. One gram of tobacco may contain between 10–20 milligrams of nicotine, enough to elicit a pharmacological effect. Smaller amounts may be delivered via nicotine gums and patches. Nicotine reaches the brain in fewer than 10 seconds via cigarette smoking, and in up to 30 minutes with other delivery methods (figure 8.21).

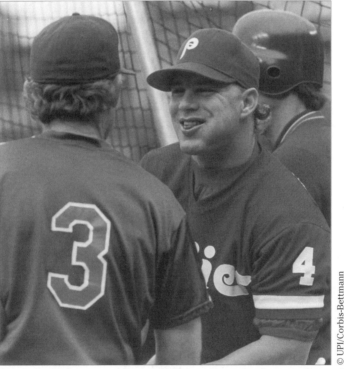

Figure 8.21 Some athletes may chew smokeless tobacco for the stimulating effect of nicotine.

Sports Performance Factor

Mental strength and physical power. Nicotine has been studied primarily in attempts to enhance various sports performance factors that may benefit from a supplemental stimulant effect. As a stimulant, nicotine also might influence all forms of physical power.

Theory

Nicotine, as a stimulant drug, may influence the brain in several ways. Nicotine may be theorized to improve neural functions such as reaction time, visual acuity, and vigilance, all factors that may enhance performance in perceptual-motor activities, such as baseball. Additionally, nicotine may elicit a sympathomimetic effect throughout the body, including the cardiovascular, respiratory, and muscular systems, responses that could enhance anaerobic and aerobic endurance capacity.

Effectiveness

The effects of nicotine on physical performance have been studied through the use of acute cigarette smoking or smokeless tobacco. The research findings are equivocal, but generally do not support an ergogenic effect of nicotine on reaction time, movement time, strength, or anaerobic and aerobic endurance. Nevertheless, some research suggests nicotine may enhance performance in tests of central nervous system arousal, such as visual and auditory reactivity. If true, these effects could enhance performance in sports requiring processing of rapidly changing stimuli, such as baseball and tennis. Conversely, some research indicates nicotine may impair hand steadiness, which could have an adverse effect in these two sports.

Safety

Nicotine may be safe if used infrequently, but may cause heartbeat irregularity in some people. Nicotine use is habit-forming; frequent use might contribute to serious health problems. Chronic cigarette smoking causes several major diseases, including heart disease, chronic obstructive lung disease, and lung cancer. Chronic use of smokeless tobacco causes oral leukoplakic lesions near the site where the tobacco is held, which may develop into oral cancer. Nicotine gums and patches in decreasing strengths may be an effective means to cease use of cigarettes or smokeless tobacco.

Legal and Ethical Aspects

Although the International Olympic Committee bans the use of stimulants, nicotine is not included in the specific list of prohibited agents, possibly because it is used worldwide as a social drug and generally has not been found to possess ergogenic qualities. Nonetheless, use of nicotine in attempts to enhance sports performance would appear to be unethical because of conflict with IOC anti-doping legislation, i.e., consuming a substance with the intent of artificially and unfairly enhancing sports performance.

Recommendations

Although legal, and safe if used only occasionally, nicotine has not been shown to be an effective ergogenic for most sports performance factors. However, many baseball players routinely use smokeless tobacco, possibly for an ergogenic effect related to enhanced central nervous system arousal. Nevertheless, oral health risks associated with chronic use of smokeless tobacco precludes recommendation of smokeless tobacco as a sports ergogenic. If future research shows nicotine to be an effective ergogenic for specific sports performance factors, use of nicotine gum or patches would be the safest approach. However, as noted above, the use of nicotine as a sports ergogenic might be considered an ethical violation.

Omega-3 Fatty Acids

Classification and Usage

Omega-3 fatty acids may be classified as a nutritional sports ergogenic. Omega-3 fatty acids are a special class of polyunsaturated fatty acids found naturally in both plant and animal foods, primarily in fish oils. One of the primary omega-3 fatty acids is eicosapentaenoic acid, or EPA.

Commercial omega-3 fatty acid supplements are available in capsule or liquid form and may be incorporated with other nutrients in various sport bars or liquid preparations. Amounts used in research approximated 4 grams per day for several weeks.

Sports Performance Factor

Mechanical edge and physical power. Omega-3 fatty acid supplementation may be used in attempts to increase muscle mass and muscular strength, or to increase aerobic power and endurance for sport events that derive energy from the oxygen energy systems.

Theory

Omega-3 fatty acids or their metabolic byproducts, various eicosanoids that function as local hormones, may be theorized to exert an ergogenic effect in several ways. First, some eicosanoids may increase the release of human growth hormone, an anabolic hormone that may stimulate protein synthesis in the muscle, increasing muscle size and strength. Second, omega-3 fatty acids may be incorporated in the red blood cell membrane, making it less viscous and able to flow more readily in blood vessels; some eicosanoids may induce a vasodilation effect, increasing the size of the blood vessels to the muscle. Both of these effects could increase oxygen delivery to the muscle during exercise, enhancing aerobic endurance performance. Third, eicosanoids may produce anti-inflammatory effects, facilitating recuperation from intense exercise training.

Effectiveness

Omega-3 fatty acid supplementation does not appear to be an effective sports ergogenic because no reputable scientific data support a beneficial effect of supplementation on muscle size or strength, aerobic capacity or performance, or recovery from intense exercise. One well-designed study investigated the interaction effect between exercise training and omega-3 fatty acid supplementation, noting that although exercise training increases VO_2max, the supplementation provided no additional benefit.

Safety

Omega-3 fatty acid supplements are safe when consumed in small amounts to complement an otherwise healthful diet. Higher dosages may prolong bleeding time, which may be harmful to some.

Legal and Ethical Aspects

Omega-3 fatty acid supplementation is legal and ethical in conjunction with sport competition.

Recommendations

Based on the available scientific evidence, omega-3 fatty acid supplementation is not an effective sports ergogenic, and its use is not recommended.

Athletes who wish to increase their intake of EPA fatty acids should incorporate more fish in their diets, particularly salmon, sardines, mackerel, and tuna. Plant sources of other omega-3 fatty acids include canola and wheat germ oils.

Oxygen Supplementation and Breathing Enhancement

Classification and Usage

Oxygen supplementation may be classified as a physiologic sports ergogenic. Oxygen is found naturally in the air we breathe and is essential for human life. Atmospheric air contains 20.9 percent oxygen, but with special canisters we can breathe oxygen concentrations of up to 100 percent. Some sport magazines advertise oxygen canisters with face masks for athletes, weighing about 1 pound and providing enough oxygen for 3 to 20 minutes, depending on exercise intensity. They may be carried in the hand while running, or strapped to the back in sports such as cycling and rowing. Varying percentages of oxygen supplementation have been provided to athletes before, during, and after exercise to determine the effects on performance and recovery.

Several breathing procedures have been used in attempts to increase oxygen intake during exercise, including nasal bandage strips, most notably Breathe Right. Breathe Right nasal strip bandages have been used extensively by professional football players and have been advertised in popular running and cycling journals. Hyperventilation and a specific breathing pattern known as *breathplay* may be useful in some sport endeavors.

Sports Performance Factor

Physical power. Oxygen supplementation and related breathing procedures are used primarily in attempts to increase aerobic power and endurance for sport events that derive energy from the oxygen energy system, but may be used in other sports, particularly those involving intermittent high-intensity anaerobic exercise tasks with brief periods of recovery between repetitions.

Theory

Oxygen is the key element of the oxygen energy system. Because the air we breathe contains only about 20 percent oxygen, oxygen supplementation is designed to provide higher oxygen concentrations, 50 percent or more, either before, during, or after exercise.

Oxygen supplementation before exercise might delay the need to breathe, which could be important to swimmers because turning the head to breathe increases resistance to forward motion and reduces swimming speed. Oxygen supplementation during exercise could increase the amount of oxygen delivered to the muscle tissues and enhance performance in aerobic endurance events. Oxygen supplementation following high-intensity, anaerobic exercise could facilitate recovery for subsequent exercise tasks.

Spring-loaded nasal bandage strips are placed on the nose in attempts to increase the size of the nasal cavity, thus decreasing airway resistance to facilitate ventilation and delivery of oxygen to the lungs.

Breathplay is a specific breathing pattern involving a powerful exhalation followed by less forceful inhalations in attempts to increase the depth of ventilation and the delivery of oxygen to the lungs.

Effectiveness

The effectiveness of oxygen supplementation, use of the nasal airway expanders, or breathplay, will be addressed separately.

Oxygen Supplementation

Oxygen supplementation before exercise has not been shown to improve athletic performance. The blood has limited ability to store additional oxygen beyond the amount provided by atmospheric oxygen. The amount of blood in the average adult might increase the storage by 70 milliliters, an insignificant amount relative to energy production. Also, unless the athlete were able to breathe the oxygen mixture immediately prior to competition, this small amount of extra oxygen would be dissipated in less than 20 seconds of breathing normal atmospheric air.

Oxygen supplementation provided continuously during aerobic endurance exercise has been shown to improve physiologic energy production and athletic performance. When breathing pure oxygen compared to room air was studied during a standard exercise task, such as running a mile at a 6-minute pace, the oxygen supplementation resulted in a lower heart rate, decreased breathing, and lower production of lactic acid. Thus, oxygen supplementation permitted the runners to produce energy more efficiently, enabling them to run at a faster pace with the same physiological effort. A recent study with national-class rowers found that a 62 percent oxygen mixture improved $\dot{V}O_2$max by 11 percent and significantly reduced the time it took to row 2,500 meters. Other studies have shown that aerobic endurance performance is improved in a linear fashion with oxygen supplementation: The higher the percentage of oxygen in the supplement, the better the performance.

Oxygen supplementation after high-intensity exercise has not been shown to improve performance in subsequent exercise tasks. One of the more popular uses of oxygen supplementation is to attempt to facilitate recovery during breaks in competitive athletic events. For example, athletes who are able to take periodic rest breaks due to the nature of their sport have been known to use oxygen, such as track athletes between heats, or football, basketball, ice hockey, and soccer players during substitutions and time-outs. Unfortunately, several well-controlled studies do not support the value of this practice. The general design of these studies involved three phases. First, the athletes performed an exercise task comparable to those found in sports, such as a series of sprints with short rest periods. Next, the athletes rested and breathed a gas mixture from a tank of either pure oxygen or a placebo of room air. Finally, the athletes repeated the exercise task. The investigators usually were interested in whether the oxygen could facilitate recovery by removing lactic acid at a faster rate or by improving performance on the second exercise task. In none of these studies was lactic acid removal or exercise performance improved by the oxygen supplementation.

In summary, oxygen supplementation appears to be an effective sports ergogenic if administered during actual aerobic endurance performance, but will not improve performance when taken before competition or facilitate recovery when taken after exercise.

Nasal Airway Expanders

Research conducted by the manufacturers of Breathe Right indicates its use may decrease nasal airway resistance. However, there are few scientific data to support its effectiveness as a sports ergogenic. In a symposium sponsored by Breathe Right manufacturers, preliminary research findings revealed the use of the Breathe Right nasal bandage, compared to a placebo bandage, might enhance recovery between exercise bouts as measured by heart-rate recovery, particularly in subjects whose nasal passages were opened significantly by the nasal bandages. Other preliminary research with cyclists indicated an increase in oxygen consumption during recovery from intense exercise, again primarily in those whose nasal passages were opened to decrease air resistance to breathing. In general, however, the findings presented at this conference indicated that use of the Breathe Right nasal bandage did not affect ventilation or oxygen consumption during exercise, nor did it benefit repeat sprint performance. Four other independent, well-controlled studies, presented at the 1996 meeting of the American College of Sports Medicine, found no effect of the Breathe Right nasal bandage on anaerobic power production on a Wingate cycle ergometer test, ventilation or oxygen uptake during mild to moderate exercise, or ventilation and oxygen consumption during recovery from maximal exercise. In another performance study, athletes performed two sets of four 40-meter dashes with a short recovery period under four conditions: control, mouthpiece control, mouthpiece with placebo nasal bandage, and mouthpiece with the Breathe Right nasal bandage. These investigators found no ergogenic effect of the Breathe Right nasal bandage on sprint performance or on respiratory rate, oxygen saturation of the blood, or measures of psychological effort (figure 8.22).

During strenuous exercise, most athletes ventilate their lungs through mouth breathing, not nasal breathing. Additionally, in the healthy athlete, lung ventilation is not believed to be the limiting factor in delivering oxygen to the muscle tissue during exercise; cardiac output or the amount of blood pumped by the heart is likely the limiting factor.

Breathing Techniques

As noted above, oxygen supplementation may be theorized to benefit sprint swimmers because it might enable them to hold their breath

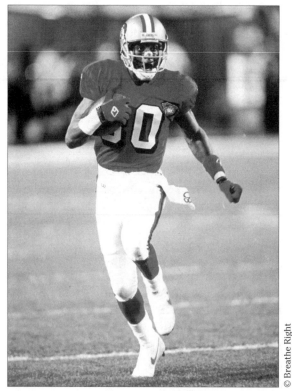

© Breathe Right

Figure 8.22 Opening up the nasal passageways with spring-loaded bandages is theorized to enhance athletic performance.

longer and not have to turn their heads to breathe, which could increase water resistance. Unfortunately, this does not appear to be practical in actual competition unless the swimmer has an oxygen tank on the starting block. Hyperventilation, or taking 5 to 10 very deep breaths just before the start, is practical and can increase breath-holding time substantially because those breaths help to lower blood levels of carbon dioxide, the main stimulus forcing you to breathe.

Some preliminary research has suggested that another breathing technique, called breathplay, might help improve the efficiency of oxygen utilization during exercise. The study was conducted with bicyclists and involved specific breathing patterns, mainly a powerful exhalation followed by less forceful inhalations. The cyclists in the study who learned the breathplay technique improved several physiological functions, such as a delay in the onset of the anaerobic threshold and a lower heart rate during a standard exercise task. They also benefited psychologically, perceiving the exercise task as less stressful. The endurance performance of the bicyclists in this study also improved with breathplay. However, the authors noted that although the results are promising, more research is needed before breathplay can be regarded as an effective sports ergogenic. Indeed, other research with rowers, varying the breathing pattern with the power and recovery phases of rowing, reported no significant effect whether or not the rowers inhaled or exhaled during either power or recovery phases, or used spontaneous breathing techniques.

Safety

The short-term use of oxygen supplementation during exercise appears to be safe. Studies have used oxygen concentrations ranging from 30 percent to 100 percent without adverse effects. Chronic use of oxygen supplementation, not likely in conjunction with sport competition, could result in oxygen toxicity. The use of the Breathe Right nasal bandage and various breathing techniques are safe.

Legal and Ethical Aspects

According to the United States Olympic Committee, use of oxygen supplementation before, during, or after exercise is legal. Although use of oxygen supplementation during exercise would appear to be illegal and unethical as an attempt to artificially improve performance, it has not been specifically prohibited by the IOC. However, various athletic governing bodies may have restrictions against the use of oxygen in conjunction with sports competition, so athletes should consult with their specific organization.

The use of the Breathe Right nasal bandage and various breathing techniques is legal and ethical.

Recommendations

Although oxygen supplementation is an effective sports ergogenic and may be safe to use during aerobic endurance exercise, carrying the additional weight may negate any ergogenic effect. Nevertheless, athletes in sports such as cycling and rowing may benefit from its use. Athletes should check with their organizations regarding legal issues and ethical concerns regarding the use of supplemental oxygen during exercise.

Based on the available scientific evidence, oxygen supplementation is not an effective sports ergogenic when used either before competition or during recovery, and hence its use is not recommended in these situations. Although oxygen supplementation under these conditions does not appear to be of any physiological value, some athletes might use it for psychological reasons. For example, NFL players may be aware that the atmospheric oxygen levels in high-altitude Denver are lower than normal and thus may believe oxygen to be ergogenic. In such cases there may be no harm in providing oxygen supplementation, as its use is legal and, in the concentrations and amounts normally used, it does not pose any medical risks. Although we cannot dismiss the potential for improved performance through the psychological placebo effect, we should also be aware of the potential for decreased performance if the placebo is not available. For example, it is the last minute of the game, the score is tied, and the key running back, who believes oxygen is ergogenic, takes a big breath from the oxygen tank and finds it empty. The running back might be affected psychologically in a negative way, and performance might suffer.

The Breathe Right nasal bandage, or similar devices, are not recommended as sports ergogenics because they have not been shown to be effective. However, their use may provide some symptomatic relief to those who experience difficulty with nasal breathing during exercise.

You may wish to experiment with different breathing patterns involving forceful exhalations and more gradual inhalations. For example, runners may exhale forcefully as one foot lands followed by inhalations on the next three foot plants; cyclists may use similar approaches in the downstroke of the bike pedal. Other endurance athletes may pattern their breathing after the mechanics of their sport. An ergogenic effect, if produced, may be psychological in nature, not physiologic. The interested reader may wish to consult *The Breathplay Approach to Whole Life Fitness,* by Ian Jackson.

Pantothenic Acid

Classification and Usage

Pantothenic acid, an essential B vitamin, may be classified as a nutritional sports ergogenic. Pantothenic acid is a water-soluble vitamin distributed widely in most plant and animal foods. The estimated safe and adequate daily dietary intake (ESADDI) for pantothenic acid is 4 to 7 milligrams per day for adults.

Pantothenic acid supplements are available individually or as part of a multivitamin/multimineral complex. Some sport drinks are fortified with pantothenic acid. Studies investigating the ergogenic effect of pantothenic acid supplementation have used dosages up to 2 grams per day for several weeks.

Sports Performance Factor

Physical power. Pantothenic acid supplementation has been studied in attempts to increase aerobic power and endurance for sport events that derive energy from the oxygen energy systems.

Theory

Pantothenic acid functions as a coenzyme for several enzymatic reactions, but one of its primary roles is to serve as a constituent of coenzyme A. Acetyl coenzyme A, or acetyl CoA, is a key metabolic intermediate in the processing of carbohydrate and fat for ATP production via the oxygen energy system in the mitochondria. Theoretically, pantothenic acid supplementation could facilitate the formation of acetyl CoA for processing through oxidative metabolic pathways, enhancing performance in prolonged aerobic endurance events.

Effectiveness

Although one brief report indicated pantothenic acid supplementation decreased lactic acid accumulation during a standardized exercise task, no performance improvement was noted. Other research with highly trained distance runners reported no significant effect of pantothenic acid supplementation on physiologic responses or run time to exhaustion in a maximal treadmill test.

Safety

Pantothenic acid is considered a safe vitamin supplement, but large doses of 10 grams or more may cause diarrhea.

Legal and Ethical Aspects

Pantothenic acid supplementation is legal and ethical in conjunction with sport competition.

Recommendations

Based on the available scientific evidence, pantothenic acid supplementation is not an effective sports ergogenic, and its use is not recommended. A pantothenic acid deficiency is almost nonexistent.

Phosphorus (Phosphate Salts)

Classification and Usage

Phosphorus, an essential mineral, may be classified as a nutritional sports ergogenic. Phosphorus is distributed widely in foods, particularly meat, seafood, eggs, milk, cheese, whole-grain products, nuts, and legumes. The Recommended Dietary Allowance is 800 milligrams for adults and 1,200 milligrams for those aged 11 to 25.

Phosphorus supplements are available as phosphate salts such as sodium, potassium, or calcium phosphate. Commercial forms targeted to athletes include Stim-O-Stam and PhosFuel. Dosages used in research approximated 4 grams per day for 3 to 6 days, usually given in four 1-gram doses over the course of the day. Sodium phosphate was most commonly used.

Sports Performance Factor

Physical power. Phosphate salts have been studied in attempts to enhance physical power in sport events that derive energy from all three human energy systems, but primarily aerobic power and endurance from the oxygen energy system.

Theory

Phosphate salts in both inorganic and organic forms play important roles in human metabolism, particularly as related to sport performance. They may influence all three human energy systems. Phosphates are part of ATP and CP, the sources of energy for the ATP-CP energy system. As intracellular buffers, phosphates may enhance the lactic acid energy system by buffering lactic acid produced during exercise. Phosphates are essential for vitamin activity and glucose utilization in aerobic exercise, producing energy via the oxygen energy system.

The theory that has received the most research attention involves the role of phosphate salts in the formation of 2,3-diphosphoglycerate (2,3-DPG), a compound in the red blood cells (RBC) that facilitates the release of oxygen to the tissues. Theoretically, an increased 2,3-DPG level would increase the delivery of oxygen to the muscle during exercise, enhancing performance in aerobic endurance activities (figure 8.23).

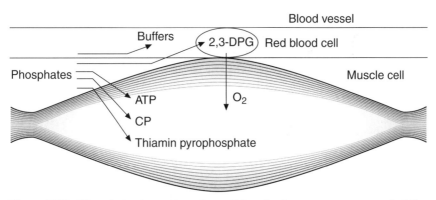

Figure 8.23 Phosphates have several possible roles in energy processes, but the most studied is its effect on 2,3-DPG as a means to release and improve aerobic endurance.

Effectiveness

There are no scientific data supporting an ergogenic effect of phosphate salt supplementation on the ATP-CP or lactic acid energy systems. Researchers at Brigham Young University reported no significant effect of Stim-O-Stam supplementation on power production, a 2- to 3-minute run to exhaustion on a treadmill, and recovery from these tests of power and anaerobic endurance. In essence, they were studying the effect of phosphate salt supplementation on the ATP-CP and lactic acid energy systems, and found no effect.

Although research findings are inconclusive, four well-controlled studies support the theory that phosphate salt supplementation may enhance function of the oxygen energy system. All four studies found that phosphate salt supplementation increased $\dot{V}O_2max$, and three reported improved performance in endurance exercise tasks, including a greater number of stages completed in a progressive treadmill running test, an increased time to exhaustion on a bicycle ergometer, and a decreased time to complete a 40-kilometer cycling test.

If phosphate salts are ergogenic, the underlying mechanism still has not been determined. Two of the studies reported an increase in 2,3-DPG levels, but the other two did not. One study found an improved heart function, with the heart pumping more blood per beat.

Two recent reviews indicated that although some research has suggested phosphate salt supplementation may be an effective sports ergogenic, more research with rigorous methodological control is needed.

Safety

Phosphate salt supplementation in amounts no larger than the RDA, and even up to 4 grams daily, appear to be safe. Excessive phosphate salt intake may cause nausea, cramps, and diarrhea. Chronic intake of phosphate salts may impair calcium balance in the body.

Legal and Ethical Aspects

Currently, phosphate salt supplementation is legal and ethical. However, consumption of 4 grams of phosphate salts per day may contravene the general meaning of the International Olympic Committee anti-doping legislation, i.e., consuming a substance in abnormal quantities with the intent of artificially and unfairly enhancing sports performance. Depending on the viewpoint of the athlete, phosphate salt supplementation may be either ethical or unethical.

Recommendations

The available research, although equivocal, provides some support for the theory, effectiveness, and safety of phosphate salt supplementation, at least in accordance with amounts recommended above, as a sports ergogenic. However, given the general tone of the IOC anti-doping legislation, the use of phosphate salt supplementation may be considered by some to be unethical.

For athletes who elect to try phosphate salt supplementation for ergogenic purposes, the regimen used in research would appear to be appropriate. The dosage was 1 gram of sodium phosphate taken four times per day, or 4 grams per day, for 3 to 4 days prior to competition. Consume the salts with adequate fluids. The last dose may be 2 to 3 hours prior to the event. As with any sports ergogenic used in conjunction with competition, experiment with its use in training beforehand.

Protein Supplements

Classification and Usage

Protein supplements may be classified as a nutritional sports ergogenic. Protein is an essential nutrient found in many foods we eat. The recommended dietary allowance for protein is .8 gram per kilogram body weight (.36 gram per pound) for adults, and .9 to 1.0 gram per kilogram (.42 to .45 gram per pound) for adolescents. A 70-kilogram adult male would need 56 grams of protein per day, easily obtainable in the typical diet.

The protein in your diet is broken down by the digestive process into 20 different amino acids. These amino acids are absorbed into your bloodstream, transported to the liver for further metabolism, and then distributed by the blood to all cells of the body for the formation of proteins specific to the functions of the different cells. We need dietary protein to provide the 20 amino acids in the appropriate amount and concentration.

Numerous commercial protein supplements available in tablet and powder forms are marketed to athletes. They normally contain high-quality milk, egg, or soy protein. Liquid dietary supplements, such as Nutrament, also contain high-quality protein. Several liquid supplements, such as GatorPro and NitroFuel, are targeted to athletes. Free-form individual amino acids also are commercially available.

Sports Performance Factor

Mechanical edge and physical power. Protein supplements have been studied primarily in attempts to increase muscle mass for enhanced strength and power or for a more aesthetic physical appearance in sports such as bodybuilding. Protein supplements may also be useful for endurance athletes as a means of replacing muscle protein used for energy during training.

Theory

Protein serves all three functions of nutrients important to exercise performance. First, protein is the primary nutrient involved in growth, development, and repair of all body tissues. Second, protein is essential for the regulation of metabolism. And third, protein may be an auxiliary source of energy.

Dietary protein, by providing amino acids, serves as the building block for muscle during resistance training. Protein also may serve as an auxiliary energy source, particularly when body stores of carbohydrate (liver and muscle glycogen) are low.

Theoretically, protein supplementation would guarantee adequate protein reserves during periods of muscle building or intense aerobic endurance exercise training.

Effectiveness

Recent well-designed protein balance studies indicate that dietary protein needs may be increased during periods of intense training, including strength training to induce muscle weight gain and intense aerobic training to increase aerobic endurance capacity. Peter Lemon, an expert on protein metabolism during exercise, recently indicated that strength-trained athletes might need about 1.4 to 1.8 grams of protein per kilogram body weight daily, while endurance athletes might need a corresponding 1.2 to 1.4 grams per kilogram.

Recent research has suggested that consumption of a protein/carbohydrate mixture immediately and 2 hours following a resistance-training workout may lead to increased secretion of both insulin and human growth hormone, two anabolic hormones that may enhance muscle growth.

However, no research is available to indicate protein supplements will enhance either muscle weight gain or aerobic endurance performance more so than an equivalent amount of normal dietary protein.

Safety

Protein supplements are derived from high-quality animal (milk and egg) or plant (soy) proteins, and are considered just as safe as the natural products. Protein supplements may have some health benefits, as they do not contain the fat or cholesterol found naturally in many high-protein foods. Conversely, they may be missing other essential nutrients found in natural protein foods.

The National Research Council does not recommend protein intake at levels greater than twice the RDA, which would be 1.6 grams per kilogram body weight for an adult. Amounts greater than this may be tolerated by most individuals, but could increase health risks for those with a diseased liver or kidney, the two organs that, respectively, catabolize protein and excrete its waste products.

Legal and Ethical Aspects

Protein supplementation is legal and ethical.

Recommendations

Athletes who consume a typical diet and enough caloric energy to maintain their body weight will obtain sufficient protein to maintain protein balance. In general, athletes involved in either strenuous strength training or strenuous aerobic endurance training may need slightly more protein in their diets. For an endurance athlete, the upper level of the recommended amount is 1.4 grams per kilogram body weight; for a strength-trained athlete, the upper level is 1.8 grams per kilogram body weight.

Let us look at some mathematics relative to protein intake. Table 8.16 presents some data relative to the daily protein requirements according to the recommendations noted. At the upper recommended level of 1.4 grams of protein per kilogram body weight, a 60-kilogram (132-pound) endurance athlete would need about 84 grams, and a 90-

TABLE 8.16
Daily Dietary Protein Intake to Meet Protein
Recommendations

	Endurance athlete	Strength athlete
Body weight, in kilograms	60	90
Recommended grams of protein per kilogram	1.4	1.8
Recommended total grams protein/day	84	162
Calories/kilogram body weight/day	44	44
Total calories/day	2,640	3,960
Recommended percent calories from protein	12 to 20	12 to 20
Calories derived from protein	316 to 528	475 to 792
Calories/gram of protein	4	4
Grams of protein consumed daily	79 to 132	119 to 198

kilogram (198-pound) strength athlete would need about 162 grams of protein per day. Obtaining these amounts of protein should pose no problem to either athlete. If each needs 44 calories per kilogram (20 calories per pound) of body weight to meet daily energy needs, then the endurance athlete will need 2,640 calories and the strength athlete will need 3,960 calories. A recommended range of daily protein intake is 12 to 20 percent of the daily caloric intake. Using these percentages, the endurance athlete could consume 316 to 528 protein calories and the strength athlete could consume 475 to 792 protein calories. Because each gram of protein equals 4 calories, the endurance athlete would get about 79 to 132 grams of protein, while the strength athlete would receive 119 to 198 grams of protein. In essence, the endurance athlete could obtain 84 grams of protein with a diet containing about 13 percent of the calories as protein, while the strength athlete could obtain 162 grams of protein with a diet containing a little over 16 percent of the calories from protein, both well within the range of 12 percent to 20 percent.

Both endurance and resistance-trained athletes may benefit from consuming a protein/carbohydrate food mixture both immediately and 2 hours following their respective exercise bouts. A recommended ratio is about 1:3 protein to carbohydrate mixture, specifically .40 gram of protein and 1.2 grams of carbohydrate per kilogram body weight. For a 70-kilogram (154-pound) athlete, this would amount to 28 grams of protein and 84 grams of carbohydrate for each of the two feedings.

The general recommendation for athletes is to obtain the protein they need through nutritious foods in their daily diets. Although protein supplements marketed for athletes may contain high-quality protein, they are usually quite expensive. Consumption of high-quality protein foods that are low in fat helps guarantee protein nutrition, and coincidentally provides many essential vitamins and minerals. Table 8.17 presents the protein content per serving of some basic food exchanges, along with the number of calories per serving; the additional calories are derived from the carbohydrate and/or fat content in the food.

High-quality protein foods are found in the milk and meat food exchanges. Unfortunately, milk and meat foods often contain substantial amounts of fat, so you must be careful to select those that contain as little fat as possible. Excellent selections include very lean meats such as fish and the white meat of chicken and turkey, lean meat

TABLE 8.17
Grams of Protein and Calories Per Serving for the Basic Food Exchanges

Skim/very-low-fat milk—8 grams protein and 90 calories per serving

1 cup skim milk	1 cup plain, low-fat yogurt

Very lean meat—7 grams protein and 35 calories per serving

1 ounce fish such as tuna (in water) or flounder
1 ounce turkey or chicken breast, no skin

Lean meat—7 grams protein and 55 calories per serving

1 ounce lean beef such as eye of round, trimmed of fat
1 ounce lean pork such as tenderloin, trimmed of fat

Starchy vegetables, legumes, breads, cereals—3 grams protein and 80 calories per serving

1/2 cup cooked or dry cereal	1 slice bread
1/2 cup cooked pasta	1 small baked potato
1/3 cup cooked rice	1/4 cup baked beans

Vegetables—2 grams protein and 25 calories per serving

1/2 cup cooked vegetables	1 cup raw vegetables

Fruits—1 gram protein and 60 calories per serving

1 small apple	1/2 banana

Note: Adapted from Exchange Lists for Meal Planning by the American Diabetes Association and American Dietetic Association, 1995, Alexandria, VA: American Diabetes Association and Chicago: American Dietetic Association Table

including lean beef and pork, egg whites, skim milk products, and legumes such as beans.

Although wholesome, natural foods are the best way to obtain dietary protein, commercial protein supplements may be recommended for some athletes. Athletes with poor eating habits and those on very-low-calorie diets (such as wrestlers and gymnasts), who need to keep caloric intake low yet obtain sufficient protein, may find protein supplements a convenient way to obtain necessary protein in the diet. However, it is important to emphasize the point that protein supplements should be used as an adjunct to an otherwise balanced nutritional plan, not as a substitute.

Riboflavin (Vitamin B$_2$)

Classification and Usage

Riboflavin, an essential vitamin also known as vitamin B$_2$, may be classified as a nutritional sports ergogenic. Riboflavin is a water-soluble vitamin found in natural foods, particularly milk, whole-grain and enriched breads and cereals, eggs, and dark-green leafy vegetables. The Recommended Dietary Allowance (RDA) for riboflavin is based on caloric intake, but approximates 1.7 milligrams for males and 1.3 milligrams for females.

Riboflavin supplements are available individually or as part of a multivitamin/multimineral complex. Some sport drinks are fortified with riboflavin. Studies investigating the ergogenic effect of riboflavin supplementation have used dosages approximating 60 milligrams per day for several weeks.

Sports Performance Factor

Physical power. Riboflavin supplementation has been studied in attempts to increase aerobic power for sport events that derive energy primarily from the oxygen energy system.

Theory

Riboflavin functions as a coenzyme for several oxidative enzyme reactions in the mitochondria. If riboflavin supplementation could enhance oxidative processes in the muscle cell, performance in aerobic endurance events theoretically could be improved.

Effectiveness

Although a riboflavin deficiency could impair sports performance, three recent reviews of the scientific literature all concluded that riboflavin supplementation has not been shown to be an effective sports ergogenic for well-nourished athletes, for it has failed to improve $\dot{V}O_2$max or the anaerobic (lactate) threshold. Riboflavin supplementation also failed to improve 50-meter swim performance, a high-power event, by elite swimmers.

Safety

Riboflavin supplements are safe and nontoxic, even in relatively large doses. Excess intake is excreted in the urine.

Legal and Ethical Aspects

Riboflavin supplementation is legal and ethical in conjunction with sport competition.

Recommendations

Based on the available scientific evidence, riboflavin supplementation is not an effective sports ergogenic and its use is not recommended.

Riboflavin need increases with increased energy expenditure, which is common with most athletes. Selecting wholesome natural foods, such as whole-grain or enriched breads and cereals, will guarantee adequate riboflavin intake for most athletes. Athletes in weight-control sports consuming very-low-calorie diets may consider taking a typical one-per-day vitamin supplement with 100 percent of the RDA for riboflavin.

Selenium

Classification and Usage

Selenium, an essential mineral, may be classified as a nutritional sports ergogenic. Selenium is found naturally in foods, particularly meat, liver, kidney, seafood, whole-grain products, and nuts. The Recommended Dietary Allowance for selenium is 70 micrograms for males and 55 micrograms for females.

Selenium supplements are available in various salt forms. Dosages used in human research approximated 100 to 180 micrograms per day for up to several months. Selenium has also been combined with other antioxidants to concoct an antioxidant cocktail.

Sports Performance Factor

Physical power. Selenium supplementation is used in attempts to increase aerobic power and endurance for sport events that derive energy primarily from the oxygen energy system.

Theory

Selenium is a cofactor for glutathione peroxidase (Gpx), a naturally occurring antioxidant enzyme in the tissues. Selenium also works closely with vitamin E, another antioxidant. Theoretically, selenium supplementation would enhance the antioxidant potential in the body, helping to prevent unwanted oxygen free radical peroxidation of lipids in red blood cell membranes and other muscle cell structures involved in the oxygen energy system. These beneficial antioxidant effects could enhance performance in prolonged aerobic endurance exercise sports.

Effectiveness

Although antioxidant supplements have not universally been shown to prevent peroxidation of lipids in cell membranes and other cell structures, some studies have shown that selenium supplementation will enhance Gpx status and reduce lipid peroxidation during prolonged aerobic exercise. Although these findings are intriguing, selenium supplementation did not improve actual physical performance, as evaluated by VO_2max or running performance of an aerobic/anaerobic nature.

Safety

Selenium supplements within RDA levels under 100 micrograms appear to be safe, but larger doses may cause adverse effects such as nausea, vomiting, abdominal pain, and unusual fatigue.

Legal and Ethical Aspects

Selenium supplementation is legal and ethical in conjunction with sport competition.

Recommendations

Based on the available scientific evidence, selenium supplementation is not an effective sports ergogenic and hence its use is not recommended. However, if foods are not selected wisely, a basic one-per-day mineral tablet containing the RDA for selenium may benefit some athletes, including (a) those who abstain from meat products, (b) those who participate in weight-control sports, (c) those involved in strenuous aerobic endurance exercise, and (d) those who live in an area with low selenium content in the soil and consume local produce.

Sodium Bicarbonate (Alkaline Salts)

Classification and Usage

Sodium bicarbonate may be classified as a physiologic sports ergogenic. Sodium bicarbonate is an alkaline salt, a part of the natural alkaline reserve in the body that helps neutralize metabolic acids.

Typical household baking soda is sodium bicarbonate. Sodium bicarbonate is marketed for athletes in gelatin capsules, often with other buffers such as sodium citrate and sodium phosphate.

Sodium bicarbonate is the most studied alkaline salt in relation to exercise performance, and the average dose used in most ergogenic studies was approximately 300 milligrams per kilogram body weight. For a 70-kilogram (154-pound) male, the total dosage would be 21 grams, about 5–6 level teaspoons, taken with 1 liter of water or other fluid 1 to 2 hours prior to exercise. The use of sodium bicarbonate is sometimes referred to as "soda loading" or "buffer boosting."

Sports Performance Factor

Physical power. Sodium bicarbonate has been studied primarily in attempts to enhance power endurance for sport events that derive energy primarily from the lactic acid energy system.

Theory

During high-intensity exercise, the accumulation of lactic acid in the muscle cell is believed to cause fatigue. The hydrogen ion released from lactic acid in the muscle cell is thought to inhibit the activity of various enzymes necessary for energy production. One theory suggests that by increasing the alkaline reserve, sodium bicarbonate supplementation will facilitate the removal of hydrogen ions from the muscle cell, reducing its acidity and delaying the onset of fatigue (figure 8.24).

Effectiveness

The ability of sodium bicarbonate to prevent fatigue of the lactic acid energy system has been studied in scores of both laboratory and field

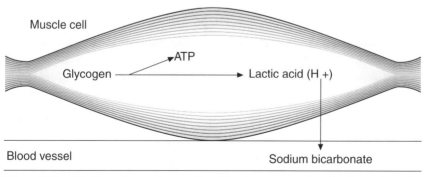

Figure 8.24 Alkaline salts, such as sodium bicarbonate, are theorized to reduce the acidity in the muscle cell by facilitating the efflux of hydrogen ions and lactic acid.

studies over the past 60 years. Various exercise protocols were used in laboratory studies, including (a) time to exhaustion in supramaximal exercise bouts at workloads greater than 100 percent $\dot{V}O_2$max, (b) time to exhaustion in the last trial of repeated bouts of supramaximal exercise interspersed with short rest periods, (c) power output in supramaximal exercise bouts ranging from 30 to 120 seconds, and (d) performance in laboratory athletic exercise tasks dependent primarily or partly on the lactic acid energy system. Field studies included running 400, 800, or 1,500 meters, swimming 100–200 meters, cycling 3–5 kilometers, rowing 500–2,000 meters, and even a 1-mile run for racehorses.

Six recent extensive reviews of these studies have concluded that sodium bicarbonate is a very effective ergogenic in events that may derive significant amounts of power from the lactic acid energy system. One of the most impressive reviews was conducted by Matson and Tran, a meta-analysis reporting that sodium bicarbonate supplementation elicited an improvement of 27 percent in laboratory tests involving time to exhaustion in supramaximal tests. In general, the majority of both laboratory and field tests have indicated sodium bicarbonate supplementation improves exercise performance in high-intensity exercise tasks ranging in duration from 45 seconds to 6 minutes, including both continuous and intermittent tasks.

Safety

In general, sodium bicarbonate supplementation is safe when taken in recommended dosages. However, some subjects may experience gastrointestinal distress, such as nausea, bloating, abdominal pain, and diarrhea. Excessive doses may cause alkalosis, which may cause muscle spasms or heart arrhythmias.

Legal and Ethical Aspects

Sodium bicarbonate is currently legal for use by athletes. However, sodium bicarbonate supplementation may contravene the general meaning of the International Olympic Committee anti-doping legislation, i.e., consuming a substance in abnormal quantities with the intent of artificially and unfairly enhancing sports performance. Depending on the viewpoint of the athlete, sodium bicarbonate supplementation may be either ethical or unethical. Detection of sodium bicarbonate utilization would be difficult with current drug-testing protocols. The urine would be alkaline, but vegetarian diets also might make the urine alkaline.

It is interesting to note that in some countries, notably Australia, supplementation of sodium bicarbonate to racehorses is prohibited.

Recommendations

Sodium bicarbonate supplementation appears to be an effective sports ergogenic, may be safe if consumed in recommended amounts, and is currently legal. Whether its use is ethical or not is debatable. Some contend that the use of sodium bicarbonate for "soda loading" may be comparable to the use of glucose polymers for "carbohydrate loading," while others suggest sodium bicarbonate may be viewed as a drug or "soda doping" and comparable to "blood doping." Given its legality but questionable ethicality, the decision to use sodium bicarbonate is up to the individual athlete.

Testosterone and Human Chorionic Gonadotropin (hCG)

Classification and Usage

Testosterone and human chorionic gonadotropin (hCG) may be classified as physiological sports ergogenics. Testosterone, a steroid, is the natural male sex hormone produced endogenously by the testes. hCG , a glycoprotein, is produced in large amounts by the placenta in pregnancy. When administered to males, hCG stimulates the production of natural testosterone, which is the main focus here.

Testosterone exerts both anabolic and androgenic effects in both males and females. Anabolic effects include increases in bone density and lean muscle mass and decreases in body fat, while androgenic effects include the development of male secondary sex characteristics, such as growth of facial and body hair, deepening of the voice, and development of the reproductive organs.

The chemical structure of testosterone may be modified in attempts to maximize the anabolic effects and minimize the androgenic effects. The resulting compounds, or drugs, are referred to as anabolic/androgenic steroids (AAS) and are addressed separately as pharmacological sports ergogenics.

Testosterone may be used therapeutically for treatment of hypogonadal males or for contraceptive purposes; pharmaceutical doses are 75 to 100 milligrams and 200 to 250 milligrams per day, respectively. Testosterone may have been used for ergogenic purposes as early as the 1936 Olympic Games, and some athletes have been reported to take 1,000 milligrams or more daily for 6 weeks. Testosterone comes in both oral and injectable forms.

Amounts ranging from 260 to 600 milligrams per week for 10 to 12 weeks have been used in studies investigating the ergogenic effect of testosterone in male subjects.

Sports Performance Factor

Mechanical edge and physical power. Testosterone and hCG are used primarily to increase muscle mass and decrease body fat for enhanced strength and power, or for a more aesthetic physical appearance in sports such as bodybuilding.

Theory

Testosterone supplementation is designed to stimulate anabolic activity, primarily to increase muscle mass by stimulating the muscle cell nucleus to enhance protein formation. Additionally, androgenic effects of testosterone include increased arousal and aggressiveness, psychological effects which have been suggested to help athletes train and perform more intensely.

Effectiveness

As noted, AAS, in conjunction with an appropriate resistance-training program and diet, will increase lean muscle mass and muscular strength. Although AAS are designed to maximize the anabolic activity of testosterone, some research has indicated that the ergogenic effect of testosterone supplementation would be comparable to that of AAS.

Two very well-controlled studies have shown that testosterone injections (testosterone enanthanate) for 10 to 12 weeks would increase lean body mass, decrease body fat, and increase strength in the bench press and squat, even in normal, sedentary young men not involved in strength training. This ergogenic effect was augmented in young men who combined testosterone injections with strength training, for they gained more lean muscle mass, lost more body fat, and lifted greater amounts of weights. In one of these studies, body composition reverted to normal when the testosterone injections were stopped.

No research investigating the sport ergogenic potential of hCG has been uncovered. If its use would increase endogenous testosterone production, however, effects similar to those seen with testosterone injections might be observed.

Safety

Although AAS may be more anabolic and less androgenic than testosterone, they are more toxic, particularly the oral forms. Thus, athletes might use testosterone because it is presumed to be a safer alternative to AAS. Testosterone does not appear to be as toxic to the liver as the AAS, but excess amounts might induce similar adverse side effects including facial and body acne, premature baldness, female-like breast enlargement in males, masculinization and deepening of the voice in females, premature closure of growth centers in adolescents, increased aggressiveness and possible violent behavior, reduction of testicular size and sperm production, and hepatitis B or AIDS with use of contaminated needles. Long-term use of testosterone may increase the risk of cardiovascular disease and prostate cancer.

hCG may also be used to help prevent some of the adverse effects of prolonged testosterone and AAS use, particularly testicular shutdown and atrophy.

Legal and Ethical Aspects

Testosterone use is prohibited by the International Olympic Committee as an anabolic agent, and hCG use is prohibited as a glycoprotein hormone. Thus, the use of either is considered illegal and unethical.

Testing for use of testosterone or hCG is more involved than testing for AAS. The liver catabolism of AAS produces various metabolic byproducts that can be analyzed easily in the urine. Testosterone is not catabolized, so it appears in the urine in its natural form, indistinguishable from oral or injectable testosterone. However, the production of natural testosterone is accompanied by another natural component, epitestosterone. A normal testosterone:epitestosterone ratio (T:E) is 1:1. Taking oral or injectable testosterone does not influence epitestosterone levels, so a urinary T:E ratio of 6:1 is used as the basis for determining the use of exogenous testosterone. Many factors can influence the T:E ratio, so additional investigation is needed to confirm a 6:1 ratio as evidence of doping.

Mary Slaney, America's greatest female middle-distance runner in history, tested positive for testosterone use at the 1996 United States Olympic Trials and has subsequently been suspended by the international federation governing track and field. Slaney contested the suspension, claiming she has never used testosterone and also noting that women's T:E ratios may vary widely depending on hormonal status.

One reason athletes may use hCG instead of testosterone itself is that hCG may stimulate the formation of both testosterone and epitestosterone, keeping the T:E ratio normal. Additionally, some athletes might take epitestosterone along with testosterone to help maintain a normal T:E ratio. Although these methods can be used to circumvent a positive doping test for testosterone, other hormonal tests have been proposed to make the testing valid.

Recommendations

Although testosterone and hCG may be presumed to be effective sports ergogenics, their use is not recommended because they are illegal and unethical. Additionally, elevated testosterone levels may increase some health risks.

Thiamin (Vitamin B₁)

Classification and Usage

Thiamin, an essential vitamin also known as vitamin B_1, may be classified as a nutritional sports ergogenic. Thiamin is a water-soluble vitamin found in natural foods, particularly pork, whole-grain products, legumes, nuts, and fruits and vegetables. The Recommended Dietary Allowance (RDA) for thiamin is based on caloric intake, but is about 1.5 milligrams for males and 1.1 milligrams for females.

Thiamin supplements are available individually or as part of a multivitamin/multimineral complex. Some sport drinks are fortified with thiamin. Studies investigating the ergogenic effect of thiamin supplementation have used dosages ranging from 5 to 120 milligrams per day.

Sports Performance Factor

Physical power and mental strength. Thiamin supplementation has been studied in attempts to increase aerobic power and endurance for sport events that derive energy primarily from the oxygen energy system. Additionally, thiamin may be used in attempts to improve mental strength by inducing a calmative effect.

Theory

Thiamin functions as a coenzyme for several enzymatic reactions, including the metabolism of carbohydrate for energy production and the formation of hemoglobin for the red blood cell (RBC). If thiamin supplementation could enhance carbohydrate metabolism and hemoglobin production, performance in aerobic endurance events theoretically could be improved.

Additionally, thiamin is involved in the formation of the neurotransmitter serotonin, which may induce a sense of relaxation and decreased anxiety, factors which may improve performance in competition such as archery and pistol shooting.

Effectiveness

A number of studies have shown that a thiamin deficiency will impair aerobic performance, but thiamin supplementation to individuals who have normal vitamin status will not enhance physical performance. There are no well-controlled studies to support the effectiveness of thiamin supplementation to well-nourished individuals as a sports ergogenic. In conjunction with vitamins B_6 and B_{12}, thiamin has been shown to improve performance in pistol shooting, possibly by increasing serotonin levels in the brain.

Safety

Thiamin supplements are safe and nontoxic, even in relatively large doses. Excess intake is excreted in the urine.

Legal and Ethical Aspects

Thiamin supplementation is legal and ethical in conjunction with sport competition.

Recommendations

Based on the available scientific evidence, thiamin supplementation is not an effective sports ergogenic and its use is not recommended.

Thiamin need increases with aerobic exercise and a high carbohydrate diet, normal characteristics of endurance athletes. Selecting wholesome natural carbohydrate foods, such as whole-grain products, fruits, and vegetables will guarantee adequate thiamin intake for endurance athletes in training. Athletes in weight-control sports consuming very-low-calorie diets may consider taking a typical once-a-day vitamin supplement with 100 percent of the RDA for thiamin.

Tryptophan (L-Tryptophan)

Classification and Usage

Tryptophan (L-Tryptophan), an essential amino acid, may be classified as a nutritional sports ergogenic. Tryptophan is a natural constituent of protein, but does not exist in free form in foods we eat. The recommended dietary allowance for tryptophan is somewhat less than 250 milligrams per day, which is easily obtainable in the typical diet.

Tryptophan supplements are commercially available in tablet or powder form in various countries as L-Tryptophan, but sale of L-Tryptophan is prohibited in the United States and Canada. Amounts used in research total approximately 1,200 milligrams consumed over a 24-hour period.

Sports Performance Factor

Mental strength and physical power. Tryptophan supplementation has been studied primarily in attempts to decrease the psychological perception of discomfort or pain associated with strenuous power endurance or aerobic power exercise, most often associated with energy production from the lactic acid and oxygen energy systems.

Theory

Tryptophan is essential for the formation of serotonin, a brain neurotransmitter that is hypothesized to decrease the perception of pain. Some investigators have postulated that athletes who show the best tolerance or resistance to pain may be able to delay the onset of fatigue during high-intensity exercise. Theoretically, tryptophan supplementation may increase serotonin production, increase the tolerance to pain, and enhance performance.

Effectiveness

Several studies investigated the ergogenic potential of L-Tryptophan to enhance performance in exercise tasks dependent somewhat on a blend of power endurance and aerobic power. In a rather well-designed double-blind, placebo, crossover experiment, L-Tryptophan supplementation improved treadmill running performance by nearly 50 percent, a remarkable improvement. The subjects in this study were asked to run to exhaustion at 80 percent VO_2max (about 8.3 miles per hour at 5 percent grade), but their running performances were highly variable and only lasted an average of 5.6 to 8.6 minutes, indicating they were not highly trained athletes. Although it was a well-designed study, the training status of the subjects may have biased the results. Other investigators doubted the findings of this study and duplicated it, using highly trained runners as subjects. Their subjects ran at 100 percent VO_2max to exhaustion (9.6 miles per hour), and they lasted a little over 7 minutes. However, these investigators reported no significant effect of L-Tryptophan supplementation on performance.

L-Tryptophan supplementation does not appear to enhance prolonged aerobic endurance. Researchers in the Netherlands added moderate amounts of L-Tryptophan to a carbohydrate sport drink and reported no significant improvement in cycling time to exhaustion at 70 to 75 percent of maximal power output when compared to the carbohydrate sport drink alone. The times under both conditions were about 2 hours.

Although research findings are limited, L-Tryptophan supplementation does not appear to be an effective ergogenic for highly trained athletes.

Safety

Some subjects in these studies experienced gastrointestinal distress or skin flushing and itching, the latter possibly attributed to the conversion of L-Tryptophan to niacin, which causes such effects. L-Tryptophan has been marketed as a putative sleep aid. In 1989–1990, use of L-Tryptophan was associated with the development of a serious neuromuscular disorder, eosinophilia-myalgia syndrome (EMS) in thousands of people, resulting in 20 deaths. Although the EMS epidemic was attributed to a contaminant in a specific brand of L-Tryptophan, some medical authorities indicate that L-Tryptophan itself has not been totally absolved as the causative agent.

Legal and Ethical Aspects

L-Tryptophan use is apparently legal and ethical in those countries where it is sold, but individuals should be aware of potential health risks.

Recommendations

L-Tryptophan supplementation has not been shown to be an effective sports ergogenic and may have some associated health risks. Therefore, L-Tryptophan supplementation is not recommended for athletes.

Vanadium (Vanadyl Sulfate)

Classification and Usage

Vanadium, a nonessential mineral, may be classified as a nutritional sports ergogenic. No Recommended Dietary Allowance has been developed for vanadium because no need has been established for it in human metabolism.

Vanadium supplements are available as vanadyl salts, primarily vanadyl sulfate. Dosages used in human research approximated 60 to 100 milligrams per day for up to 12 weeks.

Sports Performance Factor

Mechanical edge and physical power. Advertisements for vanadyl salt supplements suggest they may be used primarily to increase muscle mass for enhanced strength and power or for a more aesthetic physical appearance in sports such as bodybuilding.

Theory

Animal research suggests vanadyl salts may be involved in several enzymatic reactions. Proponents theorize vanadyl salt supplementation may produce an insulin-like effect on glucose and protein metabolism, inducing an anabolic effect on muscle by inhibiting protein degradation during exercise.

Effectiveness

The anabolic effect of vanadyl salt supplementation has been extrapolated from animal research to humans, and is totally theoretical. Although some research has shown that vanadyl sulfate supplements may improve glucose status in humans with noninsulin-dependent diabetes mellitus, there are no scientific data supporting a sports ergogenic effect on body composition. In a well-controlled study, investigators from New Zealand found that vanadyl sulfate supplementation, about 40 milligrams per day, to subjects undertaking strength training for 12 weeks had no effect on body fat or lean muscle mass. The investigators also studied strength gains in four tasks, a 1-repetition and 10-repetition maximal test for both the bench press and leg extension. There were no significant effects of vanadyl sulfate on three of the tests. Although subjects taking vanadyl sulfate did gain more on the 1-repetition maximal leg extension test during the first 4 weeks of the study, the investigators suggested this might be attributed to low scores on the pretest. The investigators concluded that vanadyl sulfate supplementation was ineffective in changing body composition, and any modest performance-enhancing effect requires further investigation.

Given the limited research data regarding the ergogenic effect of vanadyl salt supplementation, more research is warranted.

Safety

Adverse side effects of vanadyl salt supplementation may include gastrointestinal distress, primarily diarrhea. Increased sleepiness was an observation in one study. Supplementation may also cause damage to both the liver and the kidney.

Legal and Ethical Aspects

Vanadyl salt supplementation is both legal and ethical.

Recommendations

Vanadyl salt supplementation is not recommended as a sports ergogenic because no scientific data support its effectiveness to favorably modify body composition and enhance performance. Moreover, excess amounts may be toxic.

Vitamin B$_6$ (Pyridoxine)

Classification and Usage

Vitamin B$_6$, an essential B vitamin also known as pyridoxine, may be classified as a nutritional sports ergogenic. Vitamin B$_6$ is a water-soluble vitamin found in natural foods, particularly those with high protein content such as meat, fish, poultry, legumes, brown rice, and whole-grain and enriched breads and cereals. The Recommended Dietary Allowance (RDA) for vitamin B$_6$ is based on protein intake, but approximates 2 milligrams for adults.

Vitamin B$_6$ supplements are available individually or as part of a multivitamin/multimineral complex. Some sport drinks are fortified with vitamin B$_6$. Vitamin B$_6$ is combined with protein or amino acids, such as arginine and ornithine, and marketed as an anabolic agent to athletes. Studies investigating the ergogenic effect of vitamin B$_6$ supplementation have used dosages of up to 50 milligrams per day for several weeks.

Sports Performance Factor

Physical power, mental strength, mechanical edge. Vitamin B$_6$ supplementation may be used in attempts to increase muscle mass and muscular strength, and to increase power endurance and aerobic power and endurance for events that derive energy from the lactic acid and the oxygen energy systems. Additionally, vitamin B_6 may be used in attempts to improve mental strength by inducing a calmative effect.

Theory

Vitamin B_6 functions as a coenzyme for over 60 enzymatic reactions. It is intimately involved in muscle protein metabolism and supplementation may stimulate the release of human growth hormone; it may be marketed as an anabolic agent for these reasons.

Vitamin B_6 also is involved in the utilization of muscle glycogen for energy production and the formation of hemoglobin for the red blood cell (RBC) and myoglobin and oxidative enzymes for the muscle cells. If vitamin B_6 supplementation could enhance these functions, performance in both anaerobic and aerobic endurance events theoretically could be improved.

Additionally, vitamin B_6 is involved in the formation of the neurotransmitter serotonin, which may induce a sense of relaxation and decreased anxiety, factors which may improve performance in competition such as archery and pistol shooting.

Effectiveness

Although a vitamin B_6 deficiency could impair sports performance, several recent reviews of the scientific literature have concluded vitamin B_6 supplementation has not been shown to be an effective sports ergogenic for well-nourished athletes. For example, vitamin B_6 supplementation has failed to increase VO_2max, peak lactate accumulation during exercise, or swimming endurance performance. However, in conjunction with thiamin and B_{12}, vitamin B_6 has been shown to improve performance in pistol shooting, possibly by increasing serotonin levels in the brain.

Safety

Vitamin B_6 supplements within the RDA appear to be safe, but chronic use of larger doses (over 100 milligrams per day) may be associated with neurological disturbances such as loss of normal sensation and an impaired walking gait.

Legal and Ethical Aspects

Vitamin B_6 supplementation is legal and ethical in conjunction with sport competition.

Recommendations

Based on the available scientific evidence, vitamin B$_6$ supplementation is not an effective sports ergogenic, and its use is not recommended.

Selecting wholesome natural foods, such as lean meats and whole-grain or enriched breads and cereals, will guarantee adequate vitamin B$_6$ intake for most athletes. Athletes in weight-control sports consuming very-low-calorie diets may consider taking a typical one-per-day vitamin supplement with 100 percent of the RDA for vitamin B$_6$.

Vitamin B$_{12}$ (Cyanocobalamin)

Classification and Usage

Vitamin B$_{12}$, an essential B vitamin also known as cyanocobalamin, may be classified as a nutritional sports ergogenic. Vitamin B$_{12}$ is a water-soluble vitamin found only in animal foods, such as meat, fish, poultry, cheese, milk, and eggs. It is not found in plant foods. The Recommended Dietary Allowance (RDA) for vitamin B$_{12}$ is 2 micrograms per day for adults.

Vitamin B$_{12}$ supplements are available individually or as part of a multivitamin/multimineral complex. Liquid forms may be injected. Some sport drinks are fortified with vitamin B$_{12}$. Vitamin B$_{12}$ is also marketed as Dibencobal, a trade name for the dibencozide coenzyme form of vitamin B$_{12}$. Studies investigating the ergogenic effect of vitamin B$_{12}$ supplementation have used dosages up to 50 milligrams per day for several weeks, but reports from the athletic world indicate some athletes have received injections amounting to 1,000 milligrams, a dose that is 500,000 times the RDA.

Sports Performance Factor

Mechanical edge, physical power, mental strength. Vitamin B$_{12}$ supplementation may be used in attempts to increase muscle mass and strength, or to increase aerobic power and endurance for sport events that derive energy from the oxygen energy systems. Additionally, vitamin B$_{12}$ may be used in attempts to improve mental strength by inducing a calmative effect.

Theory

Vitamin B$_{12}$ functions as a coenzyme involved in the synthesis of DNA, the genetic material within the cell nucleus. Because DNA directs the synthesis of proteins in the body, vitamin B_{12} supplementation may be theorized to stimulate development of muscle protein, enhancing explosive strength and high power.

Vitamin B_{12} is also needed for optimal DNA activity in regenerating red blood cells (RBCs) in the bone marrow. Theoretically, enhanced RBC formation will increase the oxygen-carrying capacity of the blood, enhancing aerobic power and endurance.

Additionally, vitamin B_{12} is involved in the formation of the neurotransmitter serotonin, which may induce a sense of relaxation and decreased anxiety, factors which may improve performance in competition such as archery and pistol shooting.

Effectiveness

Although a vitamin B_{12} deficiency could impair sports performance, several recent reviews of the scientific literature have concluded that neither vitamin B_{12} nor Dibencobol supplementation have been shown to be an effective sports ergogenic for well-nourished athletes. For example, vitamin B_{12} supplementation has failed to increase (a) physiological functions during exercise, such as heart rate responses and VO_2max, (b) muscle performance on standardized tests of strength and power; or (c) anaerobic and aerobic performance in a half-mile run and maximal test on a cycle ergometer. However, in conjunction with thiamin and vitamin B_6, vitamin B_{12} has been shown to improve performance in pistol shooting, possibly by increasing serotonin levels in the brain.

Safety

Vitamin B_{12} is considered a safe vitamin supplement, even in megadoses thousands of times the RDA, although there are no reasons to consume such amounts.

Legal and Ethical Aspects

Vitamin B_{12} supplementation is legal and ethical in conjunction with sport competition.

Recommendations

Based on the available scientific evidence, vitamin B_{12} supplementation is not an effective sports ergogenic, and hence its use is not recommended.

Ideally, most athletes should obtain adequate vitamin B_{12} through their diets by consuming a wide variety of animal foods, such as low-fat meat and milk. However, a basic one-per-day vitamin tablet with supplemental B_{12} may benefit some athletes, including (a) complete vegetarians (vegans) who abstain from all animal products, and (b) those in weight-control sports on very-low-calorie diets.

Vitamin B₁₅ (Dimethylglycine, DMG)

Classification and Usage

Vitamin B_{15} is not a vitamin, but rather a dietary supplement that may be classified as a nutritional sports ergogenic. The actual composition of commercial vitamin B_{15} supplements may vary considerably depending on the brand, but the patented form includes a mixture of calcium gluconate and N, N-dimethylglycine (DMG), an amino acid. DMG is believed to be the active ergogenic ingredient.

Vitamin B_{15} supplements are available in pill form. Researchers have used dosages approximating 200 milligrams per day for several weeks.

Sports Performance Factor

Physical power. Vitamin B_{15} supplementation has been studied in attempts to increase aerobic power and endurance for sport events that derive energy primarily from the oxygen energy system.

Theory

DMG is theorized to enhance oxidative processes within the muscle cell, although the underlying mechanism has not been determined. One reviewer suggests DMG may serve as a methyl donor to help synthesize creatine or other substances essential to muscle cell metabolism during aerobic exercise.

Effectiveness

Anecdotal reports, unauthenticated Russian studies, and several unpublished American reports have indicated that vitamin B_{15} supplementation may improve energy metabolism during exercise (primarily by decreasing lactic acid accumulation) and increase aerobic endurance capacity. Conversely, several unpublished American reports and a peer-reviewed, published scientific study have found no benefits of vitamin B_{15} supplementation on cardiovascular or metabolic responses to exercise, $\dot{V}O_2$max, or aerobic endurance capacity. These data are clearly equivocal.

The most recent review regarding the putative ergogenicity of vitamin B_{15} supplementation was published in 1982, and no studies have been reported subsequently. Based on the available data, the more well-controlled studies do not support the effectiveness of vitamin B_{15} as a sports ergogenic, but more research would be desirable if safety concerns could be satisfied.

Safety

Vitamin B_{15} supplements may contain chemicals of unknown quality. Although B_{15} supplements may be presumed to be safe, one scientist indicated that some constituents, including DMG hydrochloride, may be mutagenic (cancer-causing).

Legal and Ethical Aspects

Vitamin B_{15} supplementation is legal and ethical in conjunction with sport competition.

Recommendations

Vitamin B_{15} supplementation is not recommended. Although its effectiveness as a sports ergogenic has not been resolved, undetermined possible long-term health risks preclude a positive recommendation.

Vitamin C (Ascorbic Acid)

Classification and Usage

Vitamin C, an essential vitamin, may be classified as a nutritional sports ergogenic. Vitamin C is a water-soluble vitamin found in natural foods, particularly fruits and vegetables such as oranges, grapefruit, broccoli, and potatoes. The Recommended Dietary Allowance (RDA) for vitamin C is 60 milligrams.

Vitamin C supplements are available in a variety of forms and dosages, and are present in some sport drinks and sport bars. Dosages used in human research have ranged up to 1,000 milligrams per day for several weeks.

Sports Performance Factor

Physical power. Although vitamin C could influence several SPFs, it is used primarily in attempts to increase aerobic power and endurance for sport events that derive energy primarily from the oxygen energy system. Vitamin C has also been used in attempts to prevent some symptoms of overtraining.

Theory

Vitamin C is involved in a number of metabolic processes in the human body, including three that may be important for the optimal functioning of the oxygen energy system. Vitamin C is involved in the synthesis of epinephrine, a hormone that may help mobilize glucose and free fatty acids for aerobic energy production. Vitamin C helps to absorb dietary iron, which is needed for the formation of hemoglobin in the red blood cell. Vitamin C also is a powerful antioxidant, helping prevent cellular damage and impairment of the immune system from oxygen free radicals generated during intense aerobic exercise.

Effectiveness

Early research emanating from eastern European countries indicated that vitamin C supplementation improved physical performance. However, some reviewers indicated the improvement in performance might be attributed to the correction of a vitamin C deficiency, as fresh fruits and vegetables were not a dietary mainstay in those countries at that time. In general, two reviewers recently noted that more contemporary, well-designed studies using vitamin C supplements of up to 1,000 milligrams per day have not reported any significant ergogenic effect on a variety of aerobic exercise performance tests. Thus, the contemporary viewpoint is that vitamin C supplements do not improve performance.

Safety

Vitamin C supplementation of 100 to 200 milligrams is sufficient to saturate the body tissues and appears to be safe for most people. Higher doses may also be safe for most individuals, but may decrease the bioavailability of minerals such as copper, may cause diarrhea, may lead to the development of kidney stones in susceptible individuals, and may cause several other adverse side effects.

Legal and Ethical Aspects

Vitamin C supplementation is legal and ethical in conjunction with sport competition.

Recommendations

Based on the available scientific evidence, vitamin C supplementation is not an effective sports ergogenic and its use is not recommended.

Ideally, most athletes should obtain adequate vitamin C through their diets, selecting foods rich in vitamin C. Some research found that a vitamin C supplement of 600 milligrams per day for 3 weeks prior to an ultramarathon run reduced the symptoms of upper respiratory tract infections after the race. A diet rich in fruits and vegetables could easily provide 100 to 200 milligrams or more per day to achieve full tissue saturation, and even 600 milligrams per day in ultraendurance athletes who consume more calories daily because of their high mileage.

Vitamin C has also been combined with other antioxidants to concoct an antioxidant cocktail. Consult table 8.3 for foods rich in vitamin C.

Vitamin E

Classification and Usage

Vitamin E, an essential vitamin, may be classified as a nutritional sports ergogenic. Vitamin E is a fat-soluble vitamin distributed widely in natural foods, particularly polyunsaturated vegetable oils (corn, safflower) and margarines made from them, whole-grain products, wheat germ, and fortified breakfast cereals. Vitamin E is composed of a mixture of tocopherols, and the Recommended Dietary Allowance (RDA) is given in alpha-tocopherol equivalents (alpha-TE). One alpha-TE represents 1 milligram alpha-tocopherol or about 1.5 International Units (IU). The RDA for males is 10 alpha-TE and for females is 8 alpha-TE

Vitamin E supplements are available in capsules and the contents are usually labeled in IU. Vitamin E may also be found in antioxidant supplements and sport bars marketed to athletes. Dosages used in human research approximated 800 to 1,200 IU per day for up to 6 months.

Sports Performance Factor

Physical power. Vitamin E supplementation is used in attempts to increase aerobic power and endurance for sport events that derive energy primarily from the oxygen energy system.

Theory

Vitamin E functions as an antioxidant in cell membranes. Theoretically, vitamin E supplementation would enhance the antioxidant potential in the body, helping to prevent the peroxidation and destruction of lipids in red blood cell (RBC) membranes by oxygen free radicals. By helping to maintain the integrity of the RBC membrane, vitamin E supplementation could help maintain optimal delivery of oxygen to the muscle cell during aerobic exercise.

Effectiveness

More than a dozen studies have investigated the ergogenic potential of vitamin E supplementation under sea level conditions and, in general, have found no significant effect on physiological responses to exercise, such as VO_2max and lactic acid production, or on various tests of aerobic endurance capacity. For example, a contemporary well-designed study indicated that although vitamin E supplementation increased vitamin E levels in the body, there were no effects on VO_2max or cycling performance in national-class racing cyclists.

However, several studies conducted under high-altitude conditions have found that vitamin E supplementation increased VO_2max, improved the anaerobic (lactate) threshold, and increased cycle ergometer exercise time to exhaustion. Exercise at altitude appears to increase lipid peroxidation, so the vitamin E may have provided a protective effect. These interesting findings need to be confirmed by additional well-controlled research.

Safety

Vitamin E supplementation, even in dosages of 400 to 1,200 IU, appears to be safe, but some individuals may experience headaches, fatigue, and diarrhea. Vitamin E supplementation may also increase the risk of bleeding in those with blood clotting disorders.

Legal and Ethical Aspects

Vitamin E supplementation is legal and ethical in conjunction with sport competition.

Recommendations

Based on the available scientific evidence, vitamin E supplementation is not recommended for athletes training and competing at sea level conditions because it has not been shown to be an effective sports ergogenic.

Vitamin E supplementation may be recommended for athletes training and competing at altitude or in high-smog areas. New RBCs develop rapidly on exposure to altitude and the possible additional peroxidation with increasing ozone levels at altitude or pollutants in smog may increase the need for vitamin E and other antioxidants.

Although research is nonexistent relative to an ergogenic effect of vitamin E supplementation in smog areas, supplementation with 400 IU appears to have been helpful at altitude and is considered safe for most people.

Vitamin E has also been combined with other antioxidants to concoct an antioxidant cocktail. Consult table 8.3 for foods rich in vitamin E.

Yohimbine

Classification and Usage

Yohimbine is a dietary supplement that may be classified as a nutritional sports ergogenic. Yohimbine is derived from the bark of several trees, most notably Pausinystalia yohimbe and Corynanthe yohimbe. Commercial yohimbine supplements are available in tablet, capsule, and liquid extract form, either individually or in combination with other plant extracts or nutrients. Dosages may vary according to the manufacturer. Researchers have used dosages ranging from approximately 15 to 20 milligrams per day, usually given in four equal doses.

Sports Performance Factor

Mechanical edge and physical power. Yohimbine has been advertised primarily for increasing muscle mass and decreasing body fat for enhanced strength and power or for a more aesthetic physical appearance in sports such as bodybuilding.

Theory

Yohimbine may function as a drug. Its most predominant activity is the antagonism of alpha 2-adrenoreceptors, the overall effect being increased activity of the parasympathetic system and decreased activity of the sympathetic nervous system. However, blockage of these receptors may lead to increased levels of norepinephrine in the blood and a paradoxical stimulation effect.

Through its effect on the parasympathetic system, yohimbine has been used experimentally in the treatment of erectile disorders and other sexual difficulties. Based on these possible applications, entrepreneurs have promoted yohimbine as a means of enhancing testosterone production. Increased testosterone supplementation could stimulate anabolic activity and increase muscle mass. The paradoxical stimulation effect of yohimbine could increase metabolism, leading to a decrease in body fat.

Effectiveness

Several preliminary studies suggest yohimbine supplementation may play a role in weight control. One study indicated that acute yohimbine supplementation increased blood levels of free fatty acids and glycerol (markers for increased fat mobilization) during exercise, but fat oxidation was not measured. Another study reported that 3 weeks of yohimbine supplementation significantly increased weight loss in obese young women on a low-calorie diet, presumably attributed to enhanced sympathetic stimulation. However, body composition was not assessed to determine if the loss was body fat or muscle mass.

Currently, there are no sound scientific data indicating that yohimbine supplementation increases serum testosterone levels, increases muscle mass, or decreases body fat in healthy athletes.

Safety

Chronic ingestion of yohimbine supplements may be associated with various side effects, such as dizziness, nervousness, headache, mild tremors, nausea, or vomiting. One report noted that acute supplementation increased mean blood pressure by 16 percent, and other adverse health effects may be associated with prolonged intake of alpha 2-adrenoreceptor antagonists.

Legal and Ethical Aspects

Yohimbine supplementation as a sports ergogenic is both legal and ethical.

Recommendations

Yohimbine supplementation is not recommended as a sports ergogenic because no reputable scientific data support its effectiveness to enhance performance.

Zinc

Classification and Usage

Zinc, an essential mineral, may be classified as a nutritional sports ergogenic. Animal foods such as meat, poultry, and seafood (particularly oysters) contain substantial amounts of zinc. Whole-grain products also are good sources of zinc. The Recommended Dietary Allowance is 15 milligrams for males and 12 milligrams for females.

Zinc supplements are available commercially as zinc salts. Dosages used in research have ranged up to 135 milligrams per day.

Sports Performance Factor

Mechanical edge and physical power. Zinc supplementation has been studied primarily in attempts to increase muscle mass and physical power, particularly explosive power, high power, and power endurance.

Theory

Zinc plays a role in the function of more than 100 enzymes in the body, including enzymes involved in protein synthesis. Theoretically, zinc supplements could enhance muscle protein synthesis, increasing strength and power. Zinc also is needed for lactic acid dehydrogenase (LDH), an enzyme important to the lactic acid energy system. Enhanced LDH activity could benefit anaerobic exercise performance.

Effectiveness

Although zinc would appear to play an important role in exercise performance, it is unusual that its ergogenic potential has received little research attention. A study with untrained, middle-aged women reported that zinc supplementation improved muscular strength and endurance in some tests, but not in others. Another study reported no significant effects of either zinc supplementation or deprivation on $\dot{V}O_2$max.

In general, these limited research data do not support an ergogenic effect of zinc supplementation in trained athletes.

Safety

Zinc supplements up to the RDA appear to be safe. Supplements of 25 to 50 milligrams may interfere with the intestinal absorption of other trace minerals, such as iron and copper, while 100 milligrams or more may adversely affect the serum lipid profile, increasing harmful LDL cholesterol and decreasing beneficial HDL cholesterol. High doses may cause nausea and vomiting and interfere with optimal immune system functions.

Legal and Ethical Aspects

Zinc supplementation is legal and ethical in conjunction with sport competition.

Recommendations

In general, zinc supplementation is not recommended as a sports ergogenic for athletes because it has not been found to effectively enhance sports performance.

Ideally, most athletes should obtain adequate zinc through their diets, selecting foods rich in zinc as noted in table 8.18. If foods are not selected wisely, a basic one-per-day mineral tablet may benefit some athletes, including (a) those who abstain from meat products, and (b) those who participate in weight-control sports. It may be especially important for young, growing athletes in weight-control sports to obtain adequate zinc, for some scientists suggest a zinc deficiency

---

TABLE 8.18
Zinc Content of Common Foods in the Food Exchanges and Fast Foods

Milk
1 cup 1% fat milk = .9 milligram
1 cup nonfat yogurt = 2.2 milligrams

Meat/fish/poultry/cheese
1 ounce Swiss cheese = 1.1 milligrams
1 ounce lean steak = 1.8 milligrams
1 ounce shrimp = .4 milligram

Breads/cereals/legumes/starchy vegetables
1 slice whole-wheat bread = .4 milligram
1 cup baked beans = 3.5 milligrams
1 cup corn = .6 milligram

Vegetables
1 cup cooked broccoli = .6 milligram
1 cup cooked spinach = 1.4 milligrams

Fruits
1 banana = .2 milligram
1/4 cup raisins = .1 milligram

Fast foods
1 Burger King BK broiler = 3.2 milligrams
1 Wendy's quarter-pound hamburger = 6.3 milligrams

may be involved in abnormalities of puberty, growth, and muscular performance in young gymnasts and wrestlers. In such cases, the recommended procedure is to supplement the normal dietary zinc intake with about 10 to 15 milligrams, the normal amount found in the typical once-a-day vitamin/mineral supplement. Some breakfast cereals are fortified with 10 to 15 milligrams of zinc per serving.

Appendix A

GUIDE TO PROHIBITED SUBSTANCES AND METHODS

Using the International Olympic Committee (IOC) guidelines for prohibited substances and methods, the United States Olympic Committee (USOC) has developed a National Anti-Doping Program (NADP) to help Olympic athletes avoid doping and the associated penalties. These guidelines also have served as the basis for most other athletic governing bodies, such as the National Collegiate Athletic Association (NCAA), in the development of their regulations regarding the use of drugs in their specific sports.

The following list represents only a partial listing of prohibited substances and methods. Even when used for medical treatment, the detected presence of a prohibited substance constitutes doping. Over-the-counter medications also may contain banned substances. To check on any specific medication you may be taking, you may consult the USOC Drug Education Hotline at 800-233-0393. You should also check with your specific athletic organization, whose doping policies and procedures may differ slightly from the IOC or USOC.

List of Prohibited Classes and Methods
I. Classes of Prohibited Substances
   A. Stimulants and Related Substances

Generic name	Example
Amfepramone	Apisate
Amiphenazole	Amphisol
Amphetamine	Benzedrine
Bemegride	Megimide
Benzphetamine	Didrex
Chlorphentermine	Lucofen
Clorprenaline	Vortel
Cocaine	Methyl-Benzoylecgonine
Diethylpropion HCL	Tenuate
Ephedrine	Bronkotabs
Etafedrine	Decapryn
Fencamfamine	Phencamine
Isoetharine HCL	Bronkosol
Isoproterenol	Isuprel
Meclofenoxate	Lucidril
Mesocarbe	Mesocarb
Metaproterenol	Alupent
Methamphetamine	Desoxyn
Methylphenidate HCL	Ritalin
Nikethamide	Coramine
Pemoline	Stimul
Phendimetrazine	Phenzine
Phenmetrazine	Preludin
Pipradol	Meratran
Pyrovalerone	Centroton

   1. Over-the-Counter Medications Containing Prohibited Stimulants

Generic name	Example
Desoxyephedrine	Vicks Inhaler
Pseudoephedrine	Actifed
	Co-Tylenol
	Sudafed
	Drixoral
Phenylpropanolamine	Allerest
	Alka-Seltzer Plus

	Contac
	Dexatrim
	4-way Formula 44
	Sine-Aid
Propylhexedrine	Benzedrex Inhaler
Ephedrine	Bronkaid
	Vatronol Nose Drops
	Herbal teas and medicines containing Ma Huang
Ma Huang	Breathe Easy Herbal Decongestant Tea
	Ephedra
	Free Herbal "Energy Tablets"

2. Caffeine Products—Banned level (12 mcg/ml urine). See Table 8.5, page 150.

B. Narcotics

Generic name	Example
Alphaprodine	Nisentil
Anileridine	Leritine
Buprenorphine	Buprenex
Dextromoramide	Dimorlin
Dextropropoxyphen	Darvon
Diamorphine	Heroin
Dipipanone	Pipadone
Levorphanol	Levo-Dromoran
Methadone HCL	Dolopine
Meperidine	Demerol
Morphine	Duromorph
Nalbuphine	Nubain
Pentazocine	Talwin
Pethidine	Demerol
Phenazocine	Narphen

C. Anabolic Agents

Generic name	Example
Clostebol	Steranabol
Dihydrotestosterone	Stanolone
Fluoxymesterone	Halotestin
Mesterolone	Proviron
Metandienone	Dianabol

Metenolone	Primobolan
Methandrostenolone	Dianabol
Methyltestosterone	Android
Nandrolone	Durabolin
Norethandrolone	Nilevar
Oxandrololone	Anavar
Oxymetholone	Anadrol
Stanozolol	Winstrol
Testosterone	Delatestryl
Clenbuterol	
Growth Hormone	
Human Chorionic Gonadotrophin	

D. Diuretics

Generic name	Example
Acetazolamide	Diamox
Benzthiazide	Aquatag
Bumetanide	Bumex
Canrenone	Aldadiene
Chlortalidone	Thalitone
Diclofenamide	Fenamide
Furosemide	Lasix
Mannitol	Osmitol
Spironolactone	Alatone
Torsemide	Demadex
Triamterene	Dyrenium

E. Peptide and Glycoprotein Hormones and Analogues

Chorionic gonadotrophin (hCG-Human chorionic gonadotrophin)
Corticotrophin (ACTH)
Growth hormone (hGH, Somatotrophin)
Erythropoietin (EPO)

II. Prohibited Methods

A. Blood Doping

B. Pharmacological, Chemical, and Physical Manipulation

Urine substitution
Epitestosterone use

III. Classes of Drugs Subject to Certain Restrictions

A. Alcohol

B. Marijuana
C. Local anesthetics
D. Corticosteroids
E. Beta-Blockers
F. Specified Beta-2 Agonists

Appendix B

APPROXIMATE EQUIVALENCES OF SELECTED UNITED STATES AND SI WEIGHTS AND MEASURES

Length

1 kilometer = 1,000 meters

1 meter = 100 centimeters

1 meter = 1,000 millimeters

1 mile = 1,760 yards

1 yard = 3 feet

1 foot = 12 inches

1 kilometer = 0.62 mile

1 meter = 1.09 yards

1 meter = 3.28 feet

1 meter = 39.37 inches
1 mile = 1.61 kilometers
1 yard = 0.91 meter
1 foot = 0.31 meter
1 inch = 2.54 centimeters
1 inch = 25.4 millimeters

Mass

1 kilogram = 1,000 grams
1 gram = 1,000 milligrams
1 milligram = 1,000 micrograms
1 pound = 16 ounces
1 kilogram = 2.2 pounds
1 kilogram = 35.2 ounces
1 pound = 0.454 kilogram
1 pound = 454 grams
1 ounce = 28.4 grams

Volume

1 liter = 1,000 milliliters
1 quart = 32 fluid ounces
1 pint = 16 fluid ounces
1 liter = 1.057 quarts
1 liter = 33.8 fluid ounces
1 quart = 0.96 liter
1 quart = 954 milliliters
1 fluid ounce = 29.6 milliliters

United States kitchen measures

1 teaspoon = 1/6 ounce, 5 grams, 5 milliliters
1 tablespoon = 1/2 ounce, 14 grams, 15 milliliters
1 cup = 8 ounces, 120 milliliters
1 quart = 4 cups

REFERENCES

Chapter 1

Anderson, O. 1995. Dad, mom, and you: Do your genes determine your performances? *Running Research News*, 11 (8): 1–4.

Burfoot, A. 1992. White men can't run. *Runner's World*, 27: 89–95.

Chatterjee, S., and Laudato, M. 1995. Gender and performance in athletics. *Sociological Biology*, 42: 124–132.

Fagard, R., Bielen, E., and Amery, A. 1991. Heritability of aerobic power and anaerobic energy generation during exercise. *Journal of Applied Physiology*, 70: 357–362.

Kearney, J. 1996. Training the Olympic athlete. *Scientific American*, 274 (6): 44–55.

Matheny, F. 1995. Unlock your genetic potential. *Bicycling*, 36: 51–53.

Smith, R.A. 1992. A historical look at enhancement of performance in sport: Muscular moralists versus muscular scientists. *American Academy of Physical Education Papers*, 25: 2–11.

Chapter 2

Bucci, L. 1993. *Nutrients as ergogenic aids for sports and exercise.* Boca Raton, FL: CRC Press.

Burke, L.M., and Read, R.S. 1993. Dietary supplements in sport. *Sports Medicine*, 15: 43–65.

Clarke, K. (Ed.). 1972. *Drugs and the coach.* Washington, DC: American Alliance for Health, Physical Education, and Recreation.

Clarkson, P.M. 1996. Nutrition for improved sports performance: Current issues on ergogenic aids. *Sports Medicine*, 21: 293–401.

Ghaphery, N.A. 1995. Performance-enhancing drugs. *Sports Medicine*, 26: 433–442.

Thein, L.A., Thein, J.M., and Landry, G.L. 1995. Ergogenic aids. *Physical Therapy*, 75: 426–439.

Voy, R. 1991. *Drugs, sports, and politics.* Champaign, IL: Human Kinetics.

Wadler, G., and Hainline, B. 1989. *Drugs and the athlete*. Philadelphia: Davis.

Wagner, J.C. 1991. Enhancement of athletic performance with drugs: An overview. *Sports Medicine*, 12: 250–265.

Williams, M.H. 1996. Ergogenic aids: A means to citius, altius, fortius, and Olympic gold? *Research Quarterly for Exercise and Sport*, 67 (Supplement): S58–S64.

——. 1995. *Nutrition for fitness and sport*. Dubuque, IA: Brown & Benchmark.

——. 1995. Nutritional ergogenics in athletics. *Journal of Sports Sciences*, 13: S63–S74.

——. 1994. The use of nutritional ergogenic aids in sports: Is it an ethical issue? *International Journal of Sport Nutrition*, 4: 120–131.

——. 1992. Ergogenic and ergolytic substances. *Medicine and Science in Sports and Exercise*, 24: S344–S348.

——. 1974. *Drugs and athletic performance*. Springfield, IL: C.C. Thomas.

Wolinsky, I., and Hickson, J. 1994. *Nutrition in exercise and sport*. Boca Raton, FL: CRC Press.

Chapter 3

Cade, R., Packer, D., Zauner, C., Kaufmann, D., Peterson, J., Mars, D., Privette, M., Hommen, N., Fregly, M., and Rogers, J. 1992. Marathon running: Physiological and chemical changes accompanying late-race functional deterioration. *European Journal of Applied Physiology*, 65: 485–491.

Chu, D.A. 1996. *Explosive power and strength*. Champaign, IL: Human Kinetics.

Dintiman, G.B., and Ward, R.D. 1988. *Sport speed*. Champaign, IL: Human Kinetics.

Fitts, R.H., and Metzger, J.M. Mechanisms of muscular fatigue. 1993. In J.R. Poortmans (Ed.), *Principles of Exercise Biochemistry* (248–268). Basel: Karger.

Hawley, J.A., and Hopkins, W.G. 1995. Aerobic glycolytic and aerobic lipolytic power systems. *Sports Medicine*, 19: 240–250.

Henderson, J. 1996. *Better runs: 25 years' worth of lessons for running faster and farther*. Champaign, IL: Human Kinetics.

Knuttgen, H.G. 1995. Force, work, and power in athletic training. *Sports Science Exchange*, 8 (4): 1–6.

Kraemer, W.J., Fleck, S.J., and Evans, W.J. 1996. Strength and power training: Physiological mechanisms of adaptation. *Exercise and Sport Sciences Reviews*, 24: 363–398.

Newsholme, E.A. 1993. Basic aspects of metabolic regulation and their application to provision of energy in exercise. In J.R. Poortmans (Ed.), *Principles of Exercise Biochemistry* (51–88). Basel: Karger.

———. 1993. Application of knowledge of metabolic integration to the problem of metabolic limitations in sprints, middle distance and marathon running. In J.R. Poortmans (Ed.), *Principles of Exercise Biochemistry* (230–247). Basel: Karger.

Pavlou, K. 1993. Energy needs of the elite athlete. *World Review of Nutrition and Dietetics*, 71: 9–20.

Peterson, J.A., Bryant, C.X., and Peterson, S.L. 1995. *Strength training for women*. Champaign, IL: Human Kinetics.

Sargeant, A.J. 1994. Human power output and muscle fatigue. *International Journal of Sports Medicine*, 15: 116–121.

Skinner, J. 1992. Application of exercise physiology to the enhancement of human performance. *American Academy of Physical Education Papers*, 25: 122–130.

Terjung, R.L. 1995. Muscle adaptations to aerobic training. *Sports Science Exchange*, 8 (1): 1–4.

Thayer, R.E., Rice, C.L., Pettigrew, F.P., Noble, E.G., and Taylor, A.W. 1993. The fibre composition of skeletal muscle. In J.R. Poortmans (Ed.), *Principles of Exercise Biochemistry* (25–50). Basel: Karger.

Wilson, D.W. 1995. Energy metabolism in muscle approaching maximal rates of oxygen utilization. *Medicine and Science in Sports and Exercise*, 27: 54–59.

Zatsiorsky, V.M. 1995. *Science and practice of strength training*. Champaign, IL: Human Kinetics.

Chapter 4

Gould, D., and Udry, E. 1994. Psychological skills for enhancing performance: Arousal regulation strategies. *Medicine and Science in Sports and Exercise*, 26: 478–485.

Greenspan, M., Fitzsimmons, P., and Biddle, S. 1991. Aspects of psychology in sports medicine. *British Journal of Sports Medicine*, 25: 178–180.

Kirschenbaum, D., McCann, S., Meyers, A., and Williams, J. 1995. Roundtable: The use of sport psychology to improve sports performance. *Sports Science Exchange*, 20 (6): 1–4.

Lakie, M., Villagra, F., Bowman, I., and Wilby, R. 1995. Shooting performance is related to forearm temperature and hand tremor size. *Journal of Sports Sciences*, 13: 313–320.

Lynch, J. 1994. Think like a champion. *Runner's World*, 29 (August): 50–55.

———. 1996. Mind over miles. *Runner's World*, 31 (May): 88–94.

Meyers, A.W., Whelan, J.P., and Murphy, S.M. 1996. Cognitive behavioral strategies in athletic performance enhancement. *Progress in Behavior Modification*, 30: 137–164.

Morgan, W., and Brown, D. 1983. Hypnosis. In M. Williams, *Ergogenic Aids in Sport* (223–252). Champaign, IL: Human Kinetics.

Murphy, S. 1994. Imagery interventions in sport. *Medicine and Science in Sports and Exercise*, 26: 486–494.

Nideffer, R.M. 1992. *Psyched to win: How to master mental skills to improve your physical performance.* Champaign, IL: Human Kinetics.

Orlick, T. 1990. *In pursuit of excellence: How to win in sport and life through mental training.* Champaign, IL: Human Kinetics.

Schmidt, R.A. 1991. *Motor learning and performance.* Champaign, IL: Human Kinetics.

Sheehan, G. 1989. *Personal best.* Emmaus, PA: Rodale Press.

Suinn, R. 1986. *Seven steps to peak performance.* Toronto: Han Huber.

Weinberg, R.S., and Gould, D. 1995. *Foundations of sport and exercise psychology.* Champaign, IL: Human Kinetics.

Chapter 5

Abbott, A.V., and Wilson, D.G. 1996. *Human-powered vehicles.* Champaign, IL: Human Kinetics.

American College of Sports Medicine. 1996. ACSM Position stand: Weight loss in wrestlers. *Medicine and Science in Sports and Exercise*, 28 (6): ix–xii.

Brownell, K.D., and Rodin, J. 1994. The dieting maelstrom: Is it possible and advisable to lose weight? *American Psychologist*, 49: 781–791.

Burke, E.R. (Ed.). 1996. *High-tech cycling*. Champaign, IL: Human Kinetics.

Burke, E.R. 1995. *Serious cycling*. Champaign, IL: Human Kinetics.

Chatard, J., Senegas, X., Selles, M., Dreanot, P., and Geyssant, A. 1995. Wet suit effect: A comparison between competitive swimmers and triathletes. *Medicine and Science in Sports and Exercise*, 27: 580–586.

Cordain, L., and Kopriva, R. 1991. Wetsuits, body density, and swimming performance. *British Journal of Sports Medicine*, 25: 31–33.

Enoka, R. 1994. *Neuromechanical basis of kinesiology*. Champaign, IL: Human Kinetics.

Fogelholm, M. 1994. Effects of bodyweight reduction on sports performance. *Sports Medicine*, 18: 249–267.

Frederick, E. 1983. Extrinsic biomechanical aids. In M. Williams (Ed.), *Ergogenic Aids in Sport* (323–339). Champaign, IL: Human Kinetics.

Hay, J. 1978. *The biomechanics of sports techniques*. Englewood Cliffs, NJ: Prentice Hall.

Kyle, C.R. 1994. Energy and aerodynamics in bicycling. *Clinics in Sports Medicine*, 13: 39–73.

Kyle, C. 1986. Athletic clothing. *Scientific American*, 254: 104–110.

Morgan, D.W., Miller, T.A., Mitchell, V.A., and Craib, M.W. 1996. Aerobic demand of running shoes designed to exploit energy storage and return. *Research Quarterly for Exercise and Sport*, 67: 102–105.

Nattiv, A., and Lynch, L. 1994. The female athlete triad. *Physician and Sportsmedicine*, 22 (January): 60–68.

Nigg, B., and Anton, M. 1995. Energy aspects for elastic and viscous shoe soles and playing surfaces. *Medicine and Science in Sports and Exercise*, 27: 92–97.

Roche, A.F., Heymsfield, S.B., and Lohman, T.G. 1996. *Human body composition*. Champaign, IL: Human Kinetics.

Schenau, G., de Groot, G., Scheurs, A., Meestger, H., and de Koning, J. 1996. A new skate allowing powerful plantar flexions improves performance. *Medicine and Science in Sports and Exercise*, 28: 531–535.

Shorten, M.R. 1993. The energetics of running and running shoes. *Journal of Biomechanics*, 26 (Supplement 1): 41–45.

Starling, R.D., Costill, D.L., Trappe, T.A., Jozsi, A.C., Trappe, S.W., and Goodpaster, B.H. 1995. Effect of swimming suit design on the energy demands of swimming. *Medicine and Science in Sports and Exercise*, 27: 1086–1089.

Sturmi, J.E., and Rutecki, G.W. 1995. When competitive bodybuilders collapse: A result of hyperkalemia. *Physician and Sportsmedicine*, 23 (November): 49–53.

Sundgot-Borgen, J. 1994. Eating disorders in female athletes. *Sports Medicine*, 17: 176–188.

Viitasalo, J., Kyrolainen, H., Bosco, C., and Alen, M. 1987. Effects of rapid weight reduction on force production and vertical jumping height. *International Journal of Sports Medicine*, 8: 281–285.

Williams, K. 1985. The relationship between mechanical and physiological energy estimates. *Medicine and Science in Sports and Exercise*, 17: 317–325.

Chapter 6

Ainsworth, B.E., Haskell, W.L., Leon, A.S., Jacobs, D.R., Montoye, H.J., Sallis, J.F., and Paffenbarger, R.S. 1993. Compendium of physical activities: Classification of energy costs of human physical activities. *Medicine and Science in Sports and Exercise*, 25: 71–80.

Kluka, D.A. 1994. Visual skills related to sports performance. *Research Consortium Newsletter*, 16 (2): 3.

Maud, P.J., and Foster, C. 1995. Physiological assessment of human fitness. Champaign, IL: Human Kinetics.

Mitchell, J.H., Haskell, W.L., and Raven, P.B. 1994. Classification of sports. *Medicine and Science in Sports and Exercise*, 26: S242–S245.

Young, W., McLean, B., and Ardagna, J. 1995. Relationship between strength qualities and sprinting performance. *Journal of Sports Medicine and Physical Fitness*, 35: 13–19.

Chapter 7

Butterfield, G. 1996. Ergogenic aids: Evaluating sport nutrition products. *International Journal of Sport Nutrition*, 6: 191–197.

Catlin, D.H., and Murray, T.H. 1996. Performance-enhancing drugs, fair competition, and Olympic sport. *Journal of the American Medical Association*, 276: 231–237.

Editors, Nutrition Reviews. 1995. Dietary supplements: Recent chronology and legislation. *Nutrition Reviews*, 53 (2): 31–36.

Kleiner, S.M. 1991. Performance-enhancing aids in sport: Health consequences and nutritional alternatives. *Journal of the American College of Nutrition*, 10: 163–176.

Lightsey, D.M., and Attaway, J.R. 1992. Deceptive tactics used in marketing purported ergogenic aids. *National Strength and Conditioning Association Journal*, 14 (2): 26–31.

Philen, R.M., Ortiz, D.I., Auerbach, S.B., and Falk, H. 1992. Survey of advertising for nutritional supplements in health and bodybuilding magazines. *Journal of the American Medical Association*, 268: 1008–1011.

Pipe, A.L. 1993. Sport, science, and society: ethics in sports medicine. *Medicine and Science in Sports and Exercise*, 25: 888–900.

Scarpino, V., Arrigo, A., Benzi, G., Garattini, S., LaVecchia,C., Bernardi, L., Silvestrini, G., and Tuccimei, G. 1990. Evaluation of prevalence of "doping" among Italian athletes. *Lancet*, 336: 1048–1050.

Sherman, W.M., and Lamb, D. 1995. Introduction to the Gatorade Sports Science Institute conference on nutritional ergogenic aids. *International Journal of Sport Nutrition*, 5:Siii–Siv.

Short, S.H., and Marquart, L.F. 1993. Sports nutrition fraud. *New York State Journal of Medicine*, 93: 112–116.

Smith, D.A., and Perry, P.J. 1992. The efficacy of ergogenic agents in athletic competition. *Annals of Pharmacotherapy*, 26: 653–659.

Wagner, J.C. 1991. Enhancement of athletic performance with drugs: An overview. *Sports Medicine*, 12: 250–265.

Williams, M.H. 1994. The use of nutritional ergogenic aids in sports: Is it an ethical issue? *International Journal of Sport Nutrition*, 4: 120–131.

Chapter 8

Alcohol

American College of Sports Medicine. 1982. Position statement on the use of alcohol in sports. *Medicine and Science in Sports and Exercise*, 14 (6): ix–x.

Eichner, E.R. 1989. Ergolytic drugs. *Sports Science Exchange*, 2 (15): 1–4.

Williams, M.H. 1994. Physical activity, fitness, and substance misuse and abuse. In C. Bouchard, R. Shephard, and T. Stephens (Eds.), *Physical Activity, Fitness, and Health*. Champaign, IL: Human Kinetics.

————. 1992. Alcohol and sports performance. *Sports Science Exchange*, 4 (40): 1–4.

————. 1991. Alcohol, marijuana and beta-blockers. In D.R. Lamb and M.H. Williams (Eds.), *Ergogenics: Enhancement of Performance in Exercise and Sport* (331–372). Dubuque, IA: Brown & Benchmark.

Amphetamines

Ivy, J. 1983. Amphetamines. In M.H. Williams (Ed.), *Ergogenic Aids in Sport* (101–127). Champaign, IL: Human Kinetics.

Lombardo, J. 1986. Stimulants and athletic performance (part 1 of 2): Amphetamines and caffeine. *The Physician and Sportsmedicine*, 14 (11): 128–141.

Anabolic/androgenic steroids (AAS)

Elashoff, J.D., Jacknow, A.D., Shain, S.G., and Braunstein, G.D. 1991. Effects of anabolic-androgenic steroids on muscle strength. *Annals of Internal Medicine*, 115: 387–393.

Friedl, K.E. 1993. Effects of anabolic steroids on physical health. In C.E. Yesalis (Ed.), *Anabolic Steroids in Sport and Exercise* (89–106). Champaign, IL: Human Kinetics.

Kicman, A.T., Cowan, D.A., Myhre, L., Nilsson, S., Tomten, S., and Oftebro, H. 1994. Effect on sports drug tests of ingesting meat from steroid (methenolone)-treated livestock. *Clinical Chemistry*, 40: 2084–2087.

Lombardo, J. 1993. The efficacy and mechanisms of action of anabolic steroids. In C.E. Yesalis (Ed.), *Anabolic Steroids in Sport and Exercise* (89–106). Champaign, IL: Human Kinetics.

Melchert, R.B., and Welder, A.A. 1995. Cardiovascular effects of androgenic-anabolic steroids. *Medicine and Science in Sports and Exercise*, 27: 1252–1262.

Middleman, A.M., and DuRant, R.H. 1996. Anabolic steroid use and associated health risk behaviors. *Sports Medicine*, 21: 251–255.

Yesalis, C.E. (Ed.) 1993. *Anabolic Steroids in Sport and Exercise*. Champaign, IL: Human Kinetics.

Anabolic phytosterols

Pearl, J. 1993. Severe reaction to "natural testosterones": How safe are the ergogenic aids? *American Journal of Emergency Medicine*, 11: 188–189.

Wheeler, K. and Garleb, K. 1991. Gamma oryzanol-plant sterol supplementation. *International Journal of Sport Nutrition*, 1: 170–177.

Williams, M.H. 1993. Nutritional supplements for strength trained athletes. *Sports Science Exchange*, 6 (6): 1–6.

Antioxidants

Cooper, K.H. 1994. *Dr. Kenneth H. Cooper's antioxidant revolution.* Nashville, TN: Thomas Nelson Publishers.

Dekkers, J.C., van Doornen, L., and Kemper, H. 1996. The role of antioxidant vitamins and enzymes in the prevention of exercise-induced muscle damage. *Sports Medicine*, 21: 213–238.

Goldfarb, A. 1993. Antioxidants: Role of supplementation to prevent exercise-induced oxidative stress. *Medicine and Science in Sports and Exercise*, 25: 232–236.

Kanter, M.M. 1994. Free radicals, exercise, and antioxidant supplementation. *International Journal of Sport Nutrition*, 4: 205–220.

LeBlanc, K. 1996. Antioxidants as ergogenic aids. *American Medical Athletic Association Quarterly* 1 (1): 6-10.

Arginine, lysine and ornithine

Aldana, S.G., and Jacobson, B.H. 1993. Weight loss and amino acids. *Health Values*, 17: 36–40.

Kreider, R.B., Miriel, V., and Bertun, E. 1993. Amino acid supplementation and exercise performance. *Sports Medicine*, 16: 190–209.

Aspartates

Banister, E.W., and Cameron, B.J. 1990. Exercise-induced hyperammonemia: Peripheral and central effects. *International Journal of Sports Medicine*, 11 (Supplement 2): S129–S142.

Wesson, M., McNaughton, L., Davies, P., and Tristram, S. 1988. *Research Quarterly for Exercise and Sport*, 59: 234–239.

Williams, M.H. 1995. *Nutrition for Fitness and Sport.* Dubuque, IA: Brown & Benchmark.

Bee pollen

Geyman, J.P. 1994. Anaphylactic reaction after ingestion of bee pollen. *Journal of the American Board of Family Practitioners*, 7: 250–252.

Woodhouse, M.L., Williams, M.H., and Jackson, C.W. 1987. The effects of varying doses of orally ingested bee pollen extract upon selected performance variables. *Athletic Training*, 22: 26–28.

Beta-blockers

Williams, M.H. (1991). Alcohol, marijuana and beta-blockers. In D.R. Lamb and M.H. Williams (Eds.), *Ergogenics: Enhancement of Performance in Exercise and Sport* (331–372). Dubuque, IA: Brown & Benchmark.

Blood doping

American College of Sports Medicine. 1996. The use of blood doping as an ergogenic aid. *Medicine and Science in Sports and Exercise*, 28 (3): i–viii.

Simon, T.L. 1994. Induced erythrocythemia and athletic performance. *Seminars in Hematology*, 31: 128–133.

Spriet, L.L. 1991. Blood doping and oxygen transport. In D.R. Lamb and M.H. Williams (Eds.), *Ergogenics: Enhancement of Performance in Exercise and Sport* (213–248). Dubuque, IA: Brown & Benchmark.

Boron

Ferrando, A.A., and Green, N.R. 1993. The effect of boron supplementation on lean body mass, plasma testosterone levels, and strength in male bodybuilders. *International Journal of Sport Nutrition*, 3: 140–149.

Nielsen, F.H. 1992. Facts and fallacies about boron. *Nutrition Today*, 27 (May/June): 6–12.

Branched-chain amino acids (BCAA)

Davis, J.M. 1995. Carbohydrates, branched-chain amino acids, and endurance: The central fatigue hypothesis. *International Journal of Sport Nutrition*, 5: S29–S38.

Madsen, K., MacLean, D.A., Kiens, B., and Christensen, D. 1996. Effects of glucose and glucose plus branched-chain amino acids or placebo on bike performance over 100km. *Journal of Applied Physiology*, 81: 2644–2650.

Caffeine

Cole, K., Costill, D., Starling, R., Goodpaster, B., Trappe, S., and Fink, W. 1996. Effect of caffeine ingestion on perception of effort and subsequent work production. *International Journal of Sport Nutrition*, 6: 14–23.

Graham, T.E., Rush, J.W., and van Soeren, M.H. 1994. Caffeine and exercise: Metabolism and performance. *Canadian Journal of Applied Physiology*, 19: 111–138.

Graham, T.E., and Spriet, L.L. 1996. Caffeine and exercise performance. *Sports Science Exchange*, 9 (1): 1–5.

Lamarine, R.J. 1994. Selected health and behavioral effects related to the use of caffeine. *Journal of Community Health*, 19: 449–466.

Nehlig, A., and Debry, G. 1994. Caffeine and sport activity: A review. *International Journal of Sport Medicine*, 15: 215–223.

Spriet, L. 1995. Caffeine and performance. *International Journal of Sport Nutrition*, 5: S84–S99.

Calcium

Clarkson, P.M., and Haymes, E.M. 1995. Exercise and mineral status of athletes: Calcium, magnesium, phosphorus, and iron. *Medicine and Science in Sports and Exercise*, 27: 831–843.

Carbohydrate supplements

Coleman, E. 1994. Update on carbohydrate: Solid versus liquid. *International Journal of Sport Nutrition*, 4: 80–88.

Conley, M.S., and Stone, M.H. 1996. Carbohydrate ingestion/supplementation for resistance exercise and training. *Sports Medicine*, 21: 7–17.

Costill, D.L., and Hargreaves, M. 1992. Carbohydrate nutrition and fatigue. *Sports Medicine*, 13: 86–92.

Coyle, E.F. 1994. Fluid and carbohydrate replacement during exercise: How much and why? *Sports Science Exchange*, 7 (3): 1–6.

Guezennec, C.Y. 1995. Oxidation rate, complex carbohydrates, and exercise. *Sports Medicine*, 19: 365–372.

Hawley, J.A., Dennis, S.C., and Noakes, T.D. 1994. Carbohydrate, fluid, and electrolyte requirements of the soccer player: A review. *International Journal of Sport Nutrition*, 4: 221–236.

Carnitine (L-Carnitine)

Cerretelli, P., and Marconi, C. 1990. L-Carnitine supplementation in humans. The effects on physical performance. *International Journal of Sports Medicine*, 11: 1–14.

Kanter, M.M., and Williams, M.H. 1995. Antioxidants, carnitine, and choline as putative ergogenic aids. *International Journal of Sport Nutrition*, 5: S120–S131.

Krahenbuhl, S. 1995. Carnitine: Vitamin or doping. *Therapeutische Umschau*, 52: 687–692.

Wagenmakers, A. 1991. L-Carnitine supplementation and performance in man. *Medicine and Sport Science*, 32: 110–127.

Choline (Lecithin)

Kanter, M.M., and Williams, M.H. 1995. Antioxidants, carnitine, and choline as putative ergogenic aids. *International Journal of Sport Nutrition*, 5: S120–S131.

Spector, S.A., Jackman, M.R., Sabounjian, L.A., Sakkas, C., Landers, D.M., and Willis, W.T. 1995. Effect of choline supplementation in trained cyclists. *Medicine and Science in Sports and Exercise*, 27: 668–673.

Chromium

Lefavi, R.G., Anderson, R.A., Keith, R.E., Wilson, G.D., McMillan, J.L., and Stone, M.H. 1992. Efficacy of chromium supplementation in athletes: Emphasis on anabolism. *International Journal of Sport Nutrition*, 2: 111–112.

Mertz, W. 1993. Chromium in human nutrition: A review. *Journal of Nutrition*, 123: 626–633.

Stearns, D.M., Belbruno, J.J., and Wetterhahn, K.E. 1995. A prediction of chromium (III) accumulation in humans from chromium dietary supplements. *FASEB Journal*, 9: 1650–1657.

Clenbuterol

Caruso, J.F., Signorile, J.F., Perry, A.C., Leblanc, B., Williams, R., Clark, M., and Bamman, M. 1995. The effects of albuterol and isokinetic exercise on the quadriceps muscle group. *Medicine and Science in Sports and Exercise*, 27: 1471–1476.

Dodd, S.L., Powers, S.K., Vrabas, I.S., Criswell, D., Stetson, S., and Hussain, R. 1996. Effects of clenbuterol on contractile and biochemical properties of skeletal muscle. *Medicine and Science in Sports and Exercise*, 28: 669–676.

Norris, S.R., Petersen, S.R., and Jones, R.L. 1996. The effect of salbutamol on performance in endurance cyclists. *European Journal of Applied Physiology*, 73: 364–368.

Prather, I.D., Brown, D.E., North, P., and Wilson, J.R. 1995. Clenbuterol: A substitute for anabolic steroids? *Medicine and Science in Sports and Exercise*, 27: 1118–1121.

Spann, C., and Winter, M.E. 1995. Effect of clenbuterol on athletic performance. *Annals of Pharmacotherapy*, 29: 75–77.

Cocaine

Lombardo, J. 1986. Stimulants and athletic performance (part 2 of 2): Cocaine and nicotine. *The Physician and Sportsmedicine*, 14 (12): 85–91.

Nademanee, K. 1992. Cardiovascular effects and toxicities of cocaine. *Journal of Addictive Diseases*, 11 (4): 71–82.

Coenzyme Q_{10}

Braun, B., Clarkson, P.M., Freedson, P.S., and Kohl, R.L. 1991. Effects of coenzyme Q_{10} supplementation on exercise performance, VO_2max, and lipid peroxidation in trained cyclists. *International Journal of Sport Nutrition*, 1: 353–365.

Laaksonen, R., Fogelholm, M., Himberg, J., Laakso, J., and Salorinne, Y. 1995. Ubiquinone supplementation and exercise capacity in trained young and older men. *European Journal of Applied Physiology*, 72: 95–100.

Malm, C., Svensson, M., Sjoberg, B., Ekblom, B., and Sjodin, B. 1996. Supplementation with ubiquinone-10 causes cellular damage during intense exercise. *Acta Physiologica Scandinavica* 157:511-512.

Creatine

Balsom, P., Soderlund, K., and Ekblom, B. 1994. Creatine in humans with special reference to creatine supplementation. *Sports Medicine*, 18: 268–280.

Greenhaff, P.L. 1995. Creatine and its application as an ergogenic aid. *International Journal of Sport Nutrition*, 5: S100–S110.

Hultman, E., Soderlund, K., Timmons, J.A., Cederblad, G., and Greenhaff, P.L. 1996. Muscle creatine loading in man. *Journal of Applied Physiology*, 81: 232–237.

Maughan, R.J. 1995. Creatine supplementation and exercise performance. *International Journal of Sport Nutrition*, 5: 94–101.

Mujika, I., Chatard, J., Lacoste, L., Barale, F., and Geyssant, A. 1996. Creatine supplementation does not improve sprint performance in competitive swimmers. *Medicine and Science in Sports and Exercise*, 28: 1435–1441.

Dehydroepiandrosterone (DHEA)

New York Academy of Sciences. 1995. Deydroepiandrosterone (DHEA) and aging. *Annals of the New York Academy of Sciences*, 774: ix–xiv, 1–350.

Skerrett, P. 1996. Helpful hormone or hype. *Healthnews*, 2 (16): 1–2.

Diuretics

Viitasalo, J., Kyrolainen, H., Bosco, C., and Alen, M. 1987. Effects of rapid weight reduction on force production and vertical jumping height. *International Journal of Sport Medicine*, 8: 281–285.

Engineered foods and dietary supplements

Knuttgen, H.G. (Ed.). 1995. Is it real or is it Met-Rx™? Penn State Sports Medicine Newsletter, 3 (6): 1–2.

Ephedrine

Fitch, K. 1986. The use of anti-asthmatic drugs: Do they affect sports performance? *Sports Medicine*, 3: 136–150.

Noakes, T.D., Gilles, H., Smith, P., Evans, A., Gabriels, G., and Derman, E.W. 1995. Pseudoephedrine ingestion is without ergogenic effect during prolonged exercise. *Medicine and Science in Sports and Exercise*, 27: S204.

Sidney, K.H., and Lefcoe, N.M. 1977. The effects of ephedrine on the physiological and psychological responses to submaximal and maximal exercise in man. *Medicine and Science in Sports*, 9: 95–99.

Erythropoietin

American College of Sports Medicine. 1996. The use of blood doping as an ergogenic aid. *Medicine and Science in Sports and Exercise*, 28 (3): i–viii.

Ekblom, B., and Berglund, B. 1991. Effect of erythropoietin administration on maximal aerobic power. *Scandinavian Journal of Medicine and Science in Sports*, 1: 88–93.

Ramotar, J. 1990. Cyclists' deaths linked to erythropoietin? *Physician and Sportsmedicine* 18 (8): 48–49.

Fat supplements

Berning, J.R. 1996. The role of medium-chain triglycerides in exercise. *International Journal of Sport Nutrition*, 6: 121–133.

Clarkson, P.M. 1996. Nutrition for improved sports performance: Current issues on ergogenic aids. *Sports Medicine*, 21: 293–401.

Coyle, E.F. 1995. Fat metabolism during exercise. *Sports Science Exchange*, 8 (6): 1–6.

Sherman, W.M., and Leenders, N. 1995. Fat loading: The next magic bullet? *International Journal of Sport Nutrition*, 5: S1–S12.

Fluid supplementation

American College of Sports Medicine. 1996. Position stand: Exercise and fluid replacement. *Medicine and Science in Sports and Exercise*, 28 (1): i–vii.

Coyle, E.F., and Montain, S.J. 1992. Benefits of fluid replacement with carbohydrate during exercise. *Medicine and Science in Sports and Exercise*, 24: S324–S330.

Peters, H.P., Akkeermans, L.M., Bol, E., and Mosterd, W. 1995. Gastrointestinal symptoms during exercise. *Sports Medicine*, 20: 65–76.

Folic acid (Folate)

Herbert, V., and Dos, K.C. 1994. Folic acid and vitamin B_{12}. In M. Shils, J. Olson, and M. Shike (Eds.), *Modern Nutrition in Health and Disease* (402–425). Philadelphia: Lea & Febiger.

Ginseng

Bahrke, M.S., and Morgan, W.P. 1994. Evaluation of the ergogenic properties of ginseng. *Sports Medicine*, 18: 229–248.

Carr, C.J. 1986. Natural plant products that enhance performance and endurance. In C.J. Carr and E. Jokl (Eds.), *Enhancers of Performance and Endurance* (139–192). Hillsdale, NJ: Lawrence Erlbaum Associates.

Dowling, E.A., Redondo, D.R., Branch, J.D., Jones, S., McNabb, G., and Williams, M.H. 1996. Effect of Eleutherococcus senticosus on submaximal and maximal exercise performance. *Medicine and Science in Sport and Exercise*, 28: 482–489.

Mar, S. 1995. The "adaptogens" (part I): Can they really help your running? *Running Research News*, 11 (5): 1–5.

———. 1995. Can adaptogens help athletes reduce their risk of infections and overtraining? *Running Research News*, 11 (9): 1–7.

Glycerol

American Running and Fitness Association. 1996. Glycerol helps fluid balance. *Running & FitNews*, 14 (6): 1.

Lamb, D.R., Lightfoot, W.S., and Myhal, M. 1997. Prehydration with glycerol does not improve cycling performance vs 6% CHO-electrolyte drink. *Medicine and Science in Sports and Exercise* 29: S249.

Legwold, G. 1994. Hydration breakthrough! A sponge called glycerol boosts endurance by super-loading your body with water. *Bicycling*, 35 (7): 72–74.

Lyons, T.P., Riedesel, M.L., Meuli, L.E., and Chick, T.W. 1990. Effects of glycerol-induced hyperhydration prior to exercise in the heat on sweating and core temperature. *Medicine and Science in Sports and Exercise*, 22: 477–483.

Montner, P., Stark, D.M., Riedesel, M.L., Murata, G., Robergs, R., Timms, M., and Chick, T.W. 1996. Pre-exercise glycerol hydration improves cycling endurance time. *International Journal of Sports Medicine* 17: 27–33.

HMB (Beta-hydroxy-beta-methylbutyrate)

Nissen, S., Sharp, R., Ray, M., Rathmacher, J., Rice, D., Fuller, J., Connelly, A., and Abumrad, N. 1996. Effect of leucine metabolite β-hydroxy-β-methylbutyrate on muscle metabolism during resistance-exercise training. *Journal of Applied Physiology*, 81: 2095–2104.

Nissen, S., Panton, L., Wilhelm, R., and Fuller, J. 1996. Effect of β-hydroxy-β-methylbutyrate (HMB) supplementation on strength and body composition of trained and untrained males undergoing intense resistance training. *FASEB Journal*, 10: A287.

Human growth hormone

Kicman, A.T., and Cowan, D.A. 1992. Peptide hormones and sport: Misuse and detection. *British Medical Bulletin*, 48: 496–517.

Lombardo, J.A., Hickson, R.C., and Lamb, D.R. 1991. Anabolic/androgenic steroids and growth hormone. In D.R. Lamb and M.H. Williams (Eds.), *Ergogenics: Enhancement of Performance in Exercise and Sport* (249–284). Dubuque, IA: Brown & Benchmark.

Yarasheski, K.E. 1994. Growth hormone: Effects on metabolism, body composition, muscle mass, and strength. *Exercise and Sport Sciences Reviews*, 22: 285–312.

Inosine

Starling, R.D., Trappe, T.A., Short, K.R., Sheffield-Moore, M., Jozsi, A.C., Fink, W.J., and Costill, D.L. 1996. Effect of inosine supplementation on aerobic and anaerobic cycling performance. *Medicine and Science in Sports and Exercise*, 28: 1193–1198.

Williams, M.H., Kreider, R.B., Hunter, D.W., Somma, C.T., Shall, L.M., Woodhouse, M.L., and Rokitski, L. 1990. Effect of inosine supplementation on 3-mile treadmill run performance and VO_2peak. *Medicine and Science in Sports and Exercise*, 22: 517–522.

Iron

Clarkson, P.M., and Haymes, E.M. 1995. Exercise and mineral status of athletes: Calcium, magnesium, phosphorus, and iron. *Medicine and Science in Sports and Exercise*, 27: 831–843.

Weaver, C.M., and Rajaram, S. 1992. Exercise and iron status. *Journal of Nutrition*, 122: 782–787.

Magnesium

McDonald, R., and Keen, C.L. 1988. Iron, zinc and magnesium nutrition and athletic performance. *Sports Medicine*, 5: 171–184.

Lukaski, H.C. 1995. Micronutrients (magnesium, zinc, and copper): Are mineral supplements needed for athletes? *International Journal of Sport Nutrition*, 5: S74–S83.

Marijuana

Williams, M.H. 1991. Alcohol, marijuana and beta-blockers. In D.R. Lamb and M.H. Williams (Eds.), *Ergogenics: Enhancement of Performance in Exercise and Sport* (331–372). Dubuque, IA: Brown & Benchmark.

Williams, M.H. 1994. Physical activity, fitness, and substance misuse and abuse. In C. Bouchard, R. Shephard, and T. Stephens (Eds.), *Physical Activity, Fitness, and Health*. Champaign, IL: Human Kinetics.

Multivitamin/mineral supplements

Keith, R. 1994. Vitamins and physical activity. In I. Wolinsky and J. Hickson (Eds.), *Nutrition in Exercise and Sport* (170–175). Boca Raton, FL: CRC Press.

van der Beek, E.J. 1991. Vitamin supplementation and physical exercise performance. *Journal of Sports Sciences*, 9: 77–89.

Williams, M.H. 1989. Vitamin supplementation and athletic performance. *International Journal of Vitamin and Nutrition Research*, Supplement 30: 163–191.

Narcotic analgesics

Ward, D.S., and Nitti, G.J. 1988. The effects of sufentanin on the hemodynamic and respiratory response to exercise. *Medicine and Science in Sports and Exercise*, 20: 579–586.

Niacin

Murray, R., Bartoli, W.P., Eddy, D.E., and Horn, M.K. 1995. Physiological and performance responses to nicotinic-acid ingestion during exercise. *Medicine and Science in Sports and Exercise,* 27: 1057–1062.

Williams, M.H. 1989. Vitamin supplementation and athletic performance. *International Journal of Vitamin and Nutrition Research,* Supplement 30: 163–191.

Nicotine

Christen, A.G., McDaniel, R.K., and McDonald, J.L. (1990). The smokeless tobacco "time bomb." *Postgraduate Medicine,* 87 (7): 69–74.

Edwards, S.W., Glover, E.D., and Schroeder, K.L. 1987. The effects of smokeless tobacco on heart rate and neuromuscular reactivity in athletes and nonathletes. *The Physician and Sportsmedicine,* 15 (7): 141–146.

Krogh, D. 1991. *Smoking: The Artificial Passion.* New York: W.H. Freeman.

Symons, J.D., and Stebbins, C.L. 1996. Hemodynamic and regional blood flow responses to nicotine at rest and during exercise. *Medicine and Science in Sports and Exercise,* 28: 457–467.

Williams, M.H. 1994. Physical activity, fitness, and substance misuse and abuse. In C. Bouchard, R. Shephard, and T. Stephens (Eds.), *Physical Activity, Fitness, and Health.* Champaign, IL: Human Kinetics.

Omega-3 fatty acids

Brilla, L., and Landerholm, T. 1990. Effect of fish oil supplementation and exercise on serum lipids and aerobic fitness. *The Journal of Sports Medicine and Physical Fitness,* 30: 173–180.

Oxygen supplementation and breathing enhancement

Bean, D. (1996). Nose training proves to be financial—but not physiological—success. *Running Research News,* 12 (6): 10–11.

Papanek, P.E., Young, C.C., Kellner, N.A., Lachacz, J.G., and Sprado, A. 1996. The effects of an external nasal dilator (Breathe Right) on anaerobic sprint performance. *Medicine and Science in Sports and Exercise,* 28: S182.

Welch, H. 1987. Effects of hypoxia and hyperoxia on human performance. *Exercise and Sport Sciences Reviews,* 15: 191–221.

Pantothenic acid

Williams, M.H. 1989. Vitamin supplementation and athletic performance. *International Journal of Vitamin and Nutrition Research,* Supplement 30: 163–191.

Phosphate salts

Kreider, R.B. 1992. Phosphate loading and exercise performance. *Journal of Applied Nutrition*, 44: 29–49.

Tremblay, M.S., Galloway, S.D., and Sexsmith, J.R. 1994. Ergogenic effects of phosphate loading: Physiological fact or methodological fiction? *Canadian Journal of Applied Physiology*, 19: 1–11.

Protein

Chandler, R.M., Byrne, H.K., Patterson, J.G., and Ivy, J.L. 1994. Dietary supplements affect the anabolic hormones after weight-training exercise. *Journal of Applied Physiology*, 76: 839–845.

Lemon, P. 1996. Is increased dietary protein necessary or beneficial for individuals with a physically active lifestyle? *Nutrition Reviews* 54: S169-S175.

Lemon, P.W. 1995. Do athletes need more dietary protein and amino acids? *International Journal of Sport Nutrition*, 5: S39–S61.

Lemon, P.W. 1994. Protein requirement of soccer. *Journal of Sport Sciences*, 12: S17–S22.

Riboflavin (Vitamin B$_2$)

van der Beek, E.J. 1991. Vitamin supplementation and physical exercise performance. *Journal of Sports Sciences*, 9: 77–89.

Selenium

Clarkson, P.M., and Haymes, E.M. 1994. Trace mineral requirements for athletes. *International Journal of Sport Nutrition*, 4: 104–119.

Tessier, F., Margaritis, I., Richard, M., Moynot, C., and Marconnet, P. 1995. Selenium and training effects on the glutathione system and aerobic performance. *Medicine and Science in Sports and Exercise*, 27: 390–396.

Sodium bicarbonate

Bird, S.R., Wiles, J., and Robbins, J. 1995. The effect of sodium bicarbonate on 1500-m racing time. *Journal of Sports Sciences*, 13: 399–403.

Horswill, C.A. 1995. Effects of bicarbonate, citrate, and phosphate loading on performance. *International Journal of Sport Nutrition*, 5: S111–S118.

Linderman, J.K., and Gosselink, K.L. 1994. The effects of sodium bicarbonate ingestion on exercise performance. *Sports Medicine*, 18: 75–80.

Matson, L.G., and Tran, Z.V. 1993. Effects of sodium bicarbonate ingestion on anaerobic performance: A meta-analytic review. *International Journal of Sport Nutrition*, 3: 2–28.

Williams, M.H. 1992. Bicarbonate loading. *Sports Science Exchange*, 4 (36): 1–4.

Testosterone and human chorionic gonadotropin (hCG)

Bhasin, S., Storer, T., Berman, N., Callegari, C., Clevenger, B., Phillips, J., Bunnell, T., Tricker, R., Shirazi, A., and Casaburi, R. 1996. The effects of supraphysiologic doses of testosterone on muscle size and strength in normal men. *New England Journal of Medicine*, 335: 1–7.

Forbes, G.B., Porta, C.R., Herr, B.E., and Griggs, R.C. 1992. Sequence of changes in body composition induced by testosterone and reversal of changes after drug is stopped. *Journal of the American Medical Association*, 267: 397–399.

Kicman, A.T., Brooks, R.V., and Cowan, D.A. 1991. Human chorionic gonadotrophin and sport. *British Journal of Sports Medicine*, 25: 73–80.

Starka, L. 1993. Epitestosterone—A hormone or not? *Endocrine Regulation*, 27: 43–48.

Yesalis, C.E. (Ed.). 1993. *Anabolic steroids in sport and exercise.* Champaign, IL: Human Kinetics.

Thiamin (Vitamin B$_1$)

Williams, M.H. 1989. Vitamin supplementation and athletic performance. *International Journal of Vitamin and Nutrition Research*, Supplement 30: 163–191.

Tryptophan

Herbert, V. 1992. L-Tryptophan: A medicolegal case against over-the-counter marketing of supplements of amino acids. *Nutrition Today*, 27 (March): 27–30.

Stensrud, T., Ingjer, F., Holm, H., and Stromme, S. 1992. L-Tryptophan supplementation does not improve running performance. *International Journal of Sports Medicine*, 13: 481–485.

Vanadium

Fawcett, J., Farquhar, S., Walker, R., Thou, T., Lowe, G., and Goulding, A. 1996. The effect of oral vanadyl sulfate on body composition and performance in weight-training athletes. *International Journal of Sport Nutrition*, 6: 382–390.

Nielsen, F. 1994. Ultratrace minerals. In M. Shils, J. Olson, and M. Shike (Eds.), *Modern Nutrition in Health and Disease* (269–286). Philadelphia: Lea & Febiger.

Vitamin B$_6$ (Pyridoxine)

Manore, M.M. 1994. Vitamin B$_6$ and exercise. *International Journal of Sport Nutrition*, 4: 89–103.

Vitamin B$_{12}$

Herbert, V., and Dos, K.C. 1994. Folic acid and vitamin B$_{12}$. In M. Shils, J. Olson, and M. Shike (Eds.), *Modern Nutrition in Health and Disease* (402–425). Philadelphia: Lea & Febiger.

Vitamin B$_{15}$

Gray, M.E., and Titlow, L.W. 1982. B$_{15}$: Myth or miracle? *The Physician and Sportsmedicine*, 10 (1): 107–112.

Vitamin C

Gerster, H. 1989. The role of vitamin C in athletic performance. *Journal of the American College of Nutrition*, 8: 636–643.

Hemila, H. 1996. Vitamin C and common cold incidence: A review of studies with subjects under heavy physical stress. *International Journal of Sports Medicine* 17: 379-383.

Vitamin E

Kagan, V.E., Spirichev, V.B., Serbinova, E.A., Witt, E., Erin, A.N., and Packer, L. 1994. In I. Wolinsky and J. Hickson (Eds.), *Nutrition in Exercise and Sport* (185–213). Boca Raton, FL: CRC Press.

Keith, R.E. 1994. Vitamins and physical activity. In I. Wolinsky and J. Hickson (Eds.), *Nutrition in Exercise and Sport* (170–175). Boca Raton, FL: CRC Press.

Tiidus, P.M., and Houston, M.E. 1995. Vitamin E status and response to exercise training. *Sports Medicine*, 20: 12–23.

Yohimbine

Kucio, C., Jonderko, K., and Piskorska, D. 1991. Does yohimbine act as a slimming drug? *Israel Journal of Medical Sciences*, 27: 550–556.

Riley, A.J. 1994. Yohimbine in the treatment of erectile disorder. *British Journal of Clinical Practice*, 48: 133–136.

Zinc

Clarkson, P.M., and Haymes, E.M. 1994. Trace mineral requirements for athletes. *International Journal of Sport Nutrition*, 4: 104–119.

INDEX

A

adaptogens 205
adenosine triphosphate (ATP), definition of 23
aerobic endurance, definition of 34, 83
aerobic power, definition of 34, 83
agencies, for nutritional information *viii*
albuterol. *See* beta-2 agonists
alcohol 94t, 117-118
    classification and usage of 117
    effectiveness of 118
    legal and ethical aspects of 119
    recommendations for 119
    safety of 119
    sports performance factors 117
    theory of 117-118
Alka-Seltzer Plus 190
American College of Sports Medicine *viii*, 125-126, 143, 195, 201, 239
amphetamines 94t, 120-122
    classification and usage of 120
    effectiveness of 121
    legal and ethical aspects of 122
    recommendations for 122
    safety of 121-122
    sports performance factors 121
    theory of 121
anabolic/androgenic steroids (AAS) 94t, 123-128
    classification and usage of 123-124
    effectiveness of 125-126
    generic names of 124t
    health risks of 127t
    legal and ethical aspects of 126-128
    recommendations for 128
    safety of 126
    sports performance factors 125
    theory of 125
anabolic phytosterols (plant sterols) 94t, 122-123
    classification and usage of 122
    effectiveness of 123
    legal and ethical aspects of 123
    recommendations for 123
    safety of 123
    sports performance factors 123
    theory of 123
anaerobic endurance, definition of 33, 83
anaerobic glycolysis 25
Andean native people 175
antioxidants 94t, 128-131
    classification and usage of 128
    effectiveness of 129
    legal and ethical aspects of 129
    recommendations for 129-131
    safety of 129
    sports performance factors 128
    theory of 128-129
antioxidant vitamins 130t
arginine, lysine, and ornithine 94t, 131-133
    classification and usage of 131
    effectiveness of 132
    legal and ethical aspects of 133
    recommendations for 133
    safety of 132-133
    sports performance factors 132
    theory of 132
Armstrong, Lance 3
arousal
    level of 51-53
    zones of 53, 54, 54f
aspartates (aspartic acid salts) 94t, 133-135
    classification and usage of 133
    effectiveness of 134
    legal and ethical aspects of 134
    recommendations for 134-135
    safety of 134
    sports performance factors 133
    theory of 133-134
Åstrand, Per-Olaf 5
athletic abilities
    genetic potential *v*
    nature of *v*
ATP-CP energy system
    characteristics of 35t
    description of 23-24
    exercise tasks 180
    generating power 32
    generating speed 33
    generating strength 32
    illustration of 23t, 24t
    purpose of 31, 32, 33, 34
    storage of 38
Australian Institute of Sport 226
autologous transfusion. *See* blood doping
autonomic nervous system 48
avulsion fractures 50

B

Bahrke, Michael 207
Bannister, Roger 50

bee pollen 94t, 135-136
classification and usage of 136
effectiveness of 135-136
legal and ethical aspects of 136
recommendations for 136
safety of 136
sports performance factors 135
theory of 135
Benzedrine 120
beta-2 agonists 94t, 138-141
classification and usage of 138-139
effectiveness of 139-140
legal and ethical aspects of 140-141
recommendations for 141
safety of 140
sports performance factors 139
theory of 139
beta-blockers 94t, 136-138
classification and usage of 136
effectiveness of 137
legal and ethical aspects of 138
recommendations for 138
safety of 138
sports performance factors 136-137
theory of 137
beta-hydroxy-beta-methylbutyrate (HMB) 96t, 210-213
classification and usage of 210-211
effectiveness of 211-212
legal and ethical aspects of 213
recommendations for 213
safety of 212-213
sports performance factors 211
theory of 211
Beyond Training: How Athletes Enhance Performance Legally and Illegally vi, 11
Bicycling 69
biomechanical barriers, definition of 4
biomechanical sport skills
for mechanical edge 63-74
research in 63-65
biomechanics 60
The Biomechanics of Sports Techniques 65
blood doping 94t, 141-144, 193
classification and usage of 141
effectiveness of 142
legal and ethical aspects of 143
recommendations for 143-144
safety of 143
sports performance factors 141
theory of 141-142
body water loss, determination of 202
boron 94t, 144-146
classification and usage of 144
effectiveness of 144-145
food rich in 145t
legal and ethical aspects of 145
recommendations for 145-146
safety of 145
sports performance factors 144
theory of 144

Boulmerka, Hassiba 35
branched-chain amino acids (BCAA) 95t, 146-149
classification and usage of 146
effectiveness of 147-148
legal and ethical aspects of 149
recommendations for 149
safety of 149
sports performance factors 146
theory of 146-147
Breathe Right 237, 239, 240, 241, 243
The Breathplay Approach to Whole Life Fitness 243
breathing enhancement. *See* oxygen supplementation
Brigham Young University 245
Bronkotabs 190
Burfoot, Amby 209
Burke, Edmund 65
Butkus, Dick 229

C

caffeine 95t, 149-153
classification and usage of 149-150
effectiveness of 151-152
legal and ethical aspects of 152-153
products with 150t
recommendations for 153
safety of 152
sports performance factors 150
theory of 150-151
calcium 95t, 154-156
classification and usage of 154
effectiveness of 154
foods with 155t
legal and ethical aspects of 155
recommendations for 155-156
safety of 154-155
sports performance factors 154
theory of 154
Callahan, Gerry 74
carbohydrate-loading, description of 165, 165t
carbohydrates
and exercise 26-27
conversion of 27t
types of 156
carbohydrate supplementation 28
carbohydrate supplements 95t, 156-165
calories in 160t
classification and usage of 156-157
effectiveness of 158
food with 160t
intake after exercise 163-165
intake before exercise 160-161
intake during exercise 161-163
legal and ethical aspects of 159
loading of 165
recommendations for 159-160
sports performance factors 157, 158-159
theory of 157-158
types of 156

cardiovascular system, purpose of 30
carnitine (L-carnitine) 95t, 166-167
classification and usage of 166
  effectiveness of 167
  legal and ethical aspects of 168
  recommendations for 168
  safety of 168
  sports performance factors 166
  theory of 166
central nervous system, purpose of 43
chemical energy, definition of 20
choline (lecithin) 95t, 168-170
  classification and usage of 168-169
  effectiveness of 169-170
  legal and ethical aspects of 170
  recommendations for 170
  safety of 170
  sports performance factors 169
  theory of 169
chromium 95t, 170-174
  classification and usage of 170
  effectiveness of 171-172
  foods with 173t
  legal and ethical aspects of 173
  recommendations for 174
  safety of 172-173
  sports performance factors 171
  theory of 171
clenbuterol. See beta-2 agonists
cocaine 95t, 174-176
  classification and usage of 174
  effectiveness of 175
  legal and ethical aspects of 176
  recommendations for 176
  safety of 175
  sports performance factors 174
  theory of 175
coenzyme Q_{10} (CoQ$_{10}$, Ubiquinone) 95t, 176-178
  classification and usage of 176
  effectiveness of 177
  legal and ethical aspects of 178
  recommendations for 178
  safety of 177-178
  sports performance factors 176
  theory of 177
competition
  and play 1
  definition of 1
conversion charts, for weights and measures 285-286
Co-Tylenol 190
creatine 95t, 178-182
  classification and usage of 178
  effectiveness of 179-181
  legal and ethical aspects of 181
  recommendations for 182
  safety of 181
  sports performance factors 178
  theory of 178-179
creatine phosphate (CP)
  description of 23
  energy source for 33
  importance in ATP-CP energy system 38

D

Davis, J. Mark 147
dehydroepiandrosterone (DHEA) 95t, 182-184
  classification and usage of 182
  effectiveness of 183
  legal and ethical aspects of 184
  recommendations for 184
  safety of 183-184
  sports performance factors 182
  theory of 183
DeMont, Rick 192
Dexedrine 120
Dietary Supplement Health and Education Act 101-102
diuretics 95t, 184-187
  classification and usage of 184
  effectiveness of 186
  legal and ethical aspects of 187
  recommendations for 187
  safety of 186-187
  sports performance factors 184
  theory of 185-186
Dolan, Tom 74
doping
  definition of 13
  purpose of 16
doping rule, of IOC 113
Dristan 110
drive theory 51, 51f
Drugs, Sports, and Politics 109
drug-use policy, of well known organizations 17

E

efficiency, attainment of 44
Elashoff, Janet 126
electrochemical energy, role of 20
eleutherococcus senticosus. See ginseng
endurance
  aerobic 34
  anaerobic 33
  definition of 32
  power 33, 83
energy
  forms of in nature 19, 19t
  importance of 4, 20
energy efficiency, definition of 60
energy production
  genetic endowment 3
  and muscle fiber type 31-34
  and nutrients 13
  and physical power 20-34
  rate of 31
  through training 3
  within muscle cells 30
energy systems
  and ATP 22-23
  supplied by 29
  supported by 29
engineered dietary supplements 95t, 187-190
  classification and usage of 187-188

effectiveness of 189
legal and ethical aspects of 190
recommendations for 190
safety of 189
sports performance factors 188
theory of 188-189
ephedrine (sympathomimetics) 95t, 190-193
classification and usage of 190-191
effectiveness of 191-192
legal and ethical aspects of 192
recommendations for 192-193
safety of 192
sports performance factors 191
theory of 191
ergogenic, definition of *vi*, 9
ergogenic aids, definition of *vi*
Ergogenic Aids in Sports vi
ergogenics
component for sport success 99
surveys relating to 99-100
erythropoietin (EPO, rEPO) 95t, 193-196
classification and usage of 193
effectiveness of 194
legal and ethical aspects of 194-195
recommendations for 195-196
safety of 194
sports performance factors 193
theory of 193
ethics, definition of 111
exercise
and carbohydrates 26-27, 29
and fat usage 28, 29

F

fast-twitch muscle fibers
description of 22
distribution of 34-35
and energy production 31-34
fuel for 27, 29, 31
and nervous system 45
fat
and exercise 28
schematic of 28t
fatigue
caused by 37-38, 56-57
definition of 37
discussion of 38-39
and mechanical edge 79
in mental strength 56-57
sites of 38, 38f, 39, 57f
fat supplementation 95t, 196-199
classification and usage of 196
effectiveness of 197-198
legal and ethical aspects of 198
recommendations for 198-199
safety of 198
sports performance factors 196
theory of 196-197
Favre, Brett 230
Federal Trade Commission 101
Fignon, Laurent 62
Finland 132

First Amendment 102
fluid supplementation (sport drinks) 95t, 199-202
classification and usage of 199
effectiveness of 200
legal and ethical aspects of 200
recommendations for 201-202
safety of 200
sports performance factors 199
theory of 199-200
folic acid 96t, 202-204
classification and usage of 202-203
effectiveness of 203
legal and ethical aspects of 203
recommendations for 203-204
safety of 203
sports performance factors 203
theory of 203
Food and Drug Administration 102, 108, 192
Food Nutrition Information Center *viii*

G

Gatorade Sport Science Institute *viii*
genetic capacity *v*
genetic endowment
in energy production 3
in energy utilization 3
genetic potential 3
athletic abilities *v*
ginseng 96t, 204-208
classification and usage of 204
effectiveness of 206-207
forms of 204
legal and ethical aspects of 207
recommendations for 207-208
safety of 207
sports performance factors 204
theory of 205-206
glucose tolerance factor (GTF) 171
glycemic index, definition of 26
glycerol 96t, 208-210
classification and usage of 208
effectiveness of 209
legal and ethical aspects of 209-210
recommendations for 210
safety of 209
sports performance factors 208
theory of 208-209
glycerol hyperhydration, procedure for 210t
glycogen
storage of 27-28
uses of 26-28
goals
achievement of *v*
barriers for 4f
Graham, Terry 151
Greenhaff, Paul 181

H

Hay, James 65
heat energy, role of 20
HMB. *See* beta-hydroxy-beta-methylbutyrate

homologous transfusion. *See* blood doping
human forces 60
human genome project 3
human growth hormone (hGH) 96t, 213-215
    classification and usage of 213
    effectiveness of 214
    legal and ethical aspects of 215
    recommendations for 215
    safety of 214
    sports performance factors 214
    theory of 214
human nature, basics of 1

I

induced erythrocythemia. *See* blood doping
Inosine 96t, 215-217
    classification and usage of 215
    effectiveness of 216
    legal and ethical aspects of 216
    recommendations for 217
    safety of 216
    sports performance factors 215
    theory of 215-216
insulin, importance of 26
International Amateur Cycling Federation 111
International Olympic Committee *viii*, 110, 111
    doping rule of 113, 143
    guidelines for prohibited substances 279
    Medical Commission of 16-17
inverted-U theory 51, 52, 52f, 53
iron 96t, 217-220
    classification and usage of 217
    effectiveness of 218-219
    food with 220t
    legal and ethical aspects of 219
    recommendations for 219-220
    safety of 219
    sports performance factors 217
    theory of 217-218

J

Jackson, Ian 243
Johnson, Michael 78

K

Kearney, Jay 3, 82
Kensler, T. 56
King, Peter 230
Krabbe, Katrin 140

L

lactic acid energy system
    characteristics of 35t
    description of 24-25
    generating endurance 33-34
    illustration of 25t
    location of operation 29
    purpose of 31-32
Lausanne Consensus Conference on Sport Nutrition 226
LeMond, Greg 62, 217
Lycra triathlon suit 67

Lynch, Jerry 50
lysine. *See* arginine

M

magnesium 96t, 220-223
    classification and usage of 220-221
    effectiveness of 221-222
    food with 222t
    legal and ethical aspects of 222
    recommendations for 223
    safety of 222
    sports performance factors 221
    theory of 221
Ma Huang 190
marijuana 96t, 223-225
    classification and usage of 223
    effectiveness of 224
    legal and ethical aspects of 225
    recommendations for 225
    safety of 224-225
    sports performance factors 223
    theory of 223
Martens, Rainer *vi*
mechanical edge
    definition of 5, 60
    energy used 60
    and fatigue 79
    obtaining 63, 84
    sports ergogenics for 79-80, 80t
    in sports performance 62-79
    techniques for 61
    through biomechanical sport skills 63-74
    through body composition 74, 75, 78
    through body height 74
    through body type 74-75
    through body weight 74-79
    through sports equipment 69-74
    through sportswear 65-69
mechanical energy, definition of 20
mechanics, definition of 60, 62
mental barriers 50
mental imagery, illustration of 55f
mental strength
    definition of 5
    fatigue of 56-57
    nutritional sports ergogenics for 58t
    pharmacological sports ergogenics for 58t
    physiological sports ergogenics for 58t
    relaxation of 46, 48, 84
    sports ergogenics for 57-58, 58t
    stimulation of 46, 48, 83
    training for 48-50
mental toughness, building of 41, 46-58
mental training methods 54-56
mental training techniques 55t
metabolic specificity
    definition of 41
    of training 46
Metabolic Technologies, Incorporated 211
metric equivalencies 284-285
minerals, roles of 227t
mitochondria, purpose of 28

Morgan, William 207
motor control center 43f
multivitamin/mineral supplements 96t, 225-228
    classification and usage of 225-226
    effectiveness of 226, 228
    legal and ethical aspects of 228
    recommendations for 228
    roles of 227t
    safety of 228
    sports performance factors 226
    theory of 226
muscle contraction, regulation of 30
muscle energy systems. See also ATP-CP energy
        system; lactic energy system; oxygen en-
        ergy system
    characteristics of 35t
muscle glycogen, importance of 26-27
muscles
    illustration of 22f
    systems of 23-29
muscular energy, source of 25

N

narcotic analgesics 96t, 228-231
    classification and usage of 228-229
    effectiveness of 229-230
    legal and ethical aspects of 230
    recommendations for 230-231
    safety of 230
    sports performance factors 229
    theory of 229
National Agriculture Library viii
National Anti-Doping Program 279
National Basketball Association, drug-use policy
    17
National Collegiate Athletic Association viii, 17,
    279
National Federation of High School Athletic As-
    sociations viii
National Football League 230
    drug-use policy 17
National Research Council 248
natural forces 60
nervous system
    energy control by 45-46
    definition of 42
    illustration of 42f, 49f
    role of 45
    sports performance factors of 41-45
    training of 41-45
neural pathway, schematic of 42f
neuromuscular specificity
    definition of 41
    of training 45
New England Journal of Medicine 184
Newsholme, Eric 146
Newsweek 1
Newton's Second Law of Motion 62-63, 185
niacin 96t, 231-232
    classification and usage of 231
    effectiveness of 231-232
    legal and ethical aspects of 232

    recommendations for 232
    safety of 232
    sports performance factors 231
    theory of 231
nicotine 96t, 232-235
    classification and usage of 232-233
    effectiveness of 234
    legal and ethical aspects of 234
    recommendations for 234-235
    safety of 234
    sports performance factors 233
    theory of 233
Nideffer, R.M. 56
Nocera, Joseph 229
nonessential nutrients 18
nonpharmacological doping 17
nutrients
    functions of 12, 12f
    list of 14t
nutritional information, agencies for viii
nutritional sports ergogenics 12-13
    definition of 12
    list of 15t
    for mental strength 58t
    purpose of 13
Nyquil 110

O

Olympic motto 2
Olympics (1984) 143
Olympics, Atlanta (1996) 193, 195
Olympics, Australia (2000) 215
Olympics, Munich (1972) 192
omega-3 fatty acids 97t, 235-236
    classification and usage of 235
    effectiveness of 236
    legal and ethical aspects of 236
    recommendations for 236
    safety of 236
    sports performance factors 235
    theory of 235
Orlick, Terry 48, 50, 56
ornithine. See arginine
overload principle 36t
Oxford University 146
oxygen energy system
    characteristics of 35t
    description of 25-29
    fuels used for 25
    generating aerobic endurance 34
    generating aerobic power 34
    illustration of 26t
    location of operation 29
oxygen supplementation 97t, 236-243
    after exercise 239
    before exercise 238
    breathing techniques 241
    classification and usage of 236-237
    during exercise 238-239
    effectiveness of 237
    legal and ethical aspects of 241
    recommendations for 242-243

oxygen supplementation *(continued)*
  safety of 241
  sports performance factors 237
  theory of 237
  through nasal airway expanders 239-241

P

pantothenic acid 97t, 243-244
  classification and usage of 243
  effectiveness of 243
  legal and ethical aspects of 244
  recommendations for 244
  safety of 244
  sports performance factors 243
  theory of 243
perceptual-motor abilities 47t
perceptual-motor skills, components of 46, 47t
48
performance
  barriers of 4
  improvement of 5
  and nutrients 12-13
performance barriers, going beyond 9-18
pharmacological sports ergogenics
  definition of 13
  for mental strength 58t
PhosFuel 245
phosphorus (phosphate salts) 97t, 244-247
  classification and usage of 244
  effectiveness of 245
  legal and ethical aspects of 246
  recommendations for 246-247
  safety of 246
  sports performance factors 244
  theory of 244-245
physical power
  basis of 22
  definition of 5
  and energy production 20-34
  and fatigue 37-38
  training principles of 36, 36t
  using sports ergogenics 39, 40t
physical power production, requirements of
  20-22
physical power training 34-37
physiological barriers, definition of 4
physiological doping agents 17
physiological sports ergogenics 17-18
  definition of 17
  for mental strength 58t
  list of 17, 17t
Pipe, Andrew 110
placebo, definition of 102
play, and competition 1
power
  aerobic 34, 83
  definition of 32, 83
  generated by 32, 33
power endurance, definition of 33, 83
Primatene 190
principle of specificity, types of 41
Progression principle 36t

prohibited methods 282
prohibited substances
  guide to 279-282
  list of 280-282
protein supplements 97t, 247-251
  calories per serving 251t
  classification and usage of 247
  effectiveness of 248
  food with 251t
  legal and ethical aspects of 249
  protein intake 250t
  recommendations for 249-251
  safety of 248
  sports performance factors 247
  theory of 247-248
Proventil 138
psychological barriers, definition of 4
psychological sports ergogenics 50-53
  arousal of 51
  drive theory 51, 51f
  inverted-U theory 51, 52, 52f 53
  training of 50-51
Public Health Service 175

R

racer's edge *v*
Ramotar, J. E. 195
rating procedure, of sports ergogenics 115-117
relaxation, of mental strength 46, 48, 84
research considerations 103-108
  control of extraneous factors 106
  control of testing environment 106
  double-blind protocol 106
  evaluation of 106-108
  experimental treatment of 105
  learning trials of 104-105
  rationale of 103
  subject groups 105
  subjects of 103-104
  tests of 104
  use of placebo 105
  use of statistics 106
reversibility principle 36t
riboflavin (vitamin B_2) 97t, 252-253
  classification and usage of 252
  effectiveness of 252
  legal and ethical aspects of 253
  recommendations for 253
  safety of 252-253
  sports performance factors 252
  theory of 252
Roy, Bill 56
Runner's World 69

S

scientific data 106-107
  individual studies of 107
  meta-analyses of 107
  reviews of 107
Se-hoon, Chung 78
selenium 97t, 253-254
  classification and usage of 253

effectiveness of 254
legal and ethical aspects of 254
recommendations for 254
safety of 254
sports performance factors 253
theory of 253
sensory control center 43f
Serious Cycling 65
Sinex 110
SI weights and measures 284-285
Slaney, Mary 259
slow-twitch muscle fibers
  description of 22
  distribution of 34-35
  and energy production 31-34
  fuel for 27, 29, 31
  and nervous system 45
Smith, Lonnie 176
sodium bicarbonate (alkaline salts) 97t, 254-257
  classification and usage of 254
  effectiveness of 255-256
  legal and ethical aspects of 256
  recommendations for 257
  safety of 256
  sports performance factors 255
  theory of 255
sodium bicarbonate supplementation 107
specialists, in field of sports improvement 2
specificity principle 36t, 41
speed
  definition of 33, 83
  generated by 33
sport biomechanics 60
sport biomechanists, purpose of 4
sport energy, forms of 20
sport physiologists, purpose of 4
sports, definition of 1
sports achievement, improvement in 3
sport science research
  areas of 10
  increase in 10
sport scientists, importance of 2
sports equipment
  implements of 71
  for mechanical edge 69-74
  objects of 71
  vehicles of 72-74
sports ergogenics
  advertisements about 100-101
  articles about 101-102
  classification of 11-18
  definition of *vi*, 9
  effectiveness of 100-107
  ethics of 111-113
  legality of 109-110
  for mechanical edge 79-80, 80t
  for mental strength 57-58, 58t
  personal experiences 102-103
  personal testimonies about 102
  for physical power 39, 40t
  purpose of 10-11

rating of 115-278
recommendations of 113
relating to sports performance factors 94t-97t
reports about 102
reputable scientific data 106-107
research about 103-108
safety of 108-109
surveys relating to 99-100
and training techniques 11
used for 9-18
sports ergogenics. *See* individual name
sports performance
  dependency on energy production 20, 30
  enhancement of 10, 10t
  factors of 5
  improvement in 2
  and nutrients 12-13
sports performance factors 6-7, 7t
  classifications of 6-7
  for nervous system 41-45
  importance of genetics 6-7, 7t
  importance of training 6-7, 7t
  relative to mechanical edge 81, 82t, 84
  relative to mental strength 81, 82t, 83-84
  relative to physical power 81, 82t, 83
  relative to specific sports 81-84, 85t-92t, 93
  relative to sports ergogenics 81, 93, 94t-97t
sports success 5
sports training 5
sportswear
  for buoyancy 67
  for fluid resistance 66-67
  for friction 69
  for gravity 67-68
  for mechanical edge 65-69
  types of 65-66
Spriet, Lawrence 151, 153
Stim-O-Stam 245
stimulation, of mental strength 46, 48, 83
strength
  definition of 32
  explosiveness 32, 83
  generated by 32
Sudafed 110
Suinn, R. 56

T

testosterone and human chorionic gonadotro-pin (hCG) 97t, 257-260
  classification and usage of 257-258
  effectiveness of 258
  legal and ethical aspects of 259-260
  recommendations for 260
  safety of 258-259
  sports performance factors 258
  theory of 258
thiamin (Vitamin B_1) 97t, 260-262
  classification and usage of 260
  effectiveness of 261
  legal and ethical aspects of 261
  recommendations for 261

thiamin (Vitamin B₁) *(continued)*
  safety of 261
  sports performance factors 260
  theory of 260-261
Time 1
Tokyo 209
Tour de France 62, 217
trainers, importance of 2
training principles, for physical power 36t
training techniques, and sports ergogenics 11
triglycerides
  storage of 28, 28f
  types of 28
trimethylxanthine. *See* caffeine
tryptophan (L-tryptophan) 97t, 262-264
  classification and usage of 262
  effectiveness of 262-263
  legal and ethical aspects of 263
  recommendations for 263
  safety of 263
  sports performance factors 262
  theory of 262
Turner, Michael 99

U

United States Dietary Supplement Health and Education Act of 1994 108
United States Olympic Committee 109, 110, 279
  drug-use policy 17
United States Olympic Committee Drug Education Hotline *viii*, 279
United States Olympic Trials (1996) 260
United States Olympic Training Center 5
United States weights and measures 284-285
University of Virginia 148

V

vanadium (vanadyl sulfate) 97t, 264-265
  classification and usage of 264
  effectiveness of 264-265
  legal and ethical aspects of 265
  recommendations for 265
  safety of 265
  sports performance factors 264
  theory of 264
Ventolin 138
Vicks Inhaler 190
vitamin B₆ (pyridoxine) 97t, 265-267
  classification and usage of 265
  effectiveness of 266
  legal and ethical aspects of 266
  recommendations for 267
  safety of 266
  sports performance factors 265-266
  theory of 266
vitamin B₁₂ (cyanocobalamin) 97t, 267-269
  classification and usage of 267
  effectiveness of 268
  legal and ethical aspects of 268
  recommendations for 268-269

  safety of 268
  sports performance factors 267
  theory of 267-268
vitamin B₁₅ (dimethylglycine, DMG) 97t, 269-270
  classification and usage of 269
  effectiveness of 269-270
  legal and ethical aspects of 270
  recommendations for 270
  safety of 270
  sports performance factors 269
  theory of 269
vitamin C (ascorbic acid) 97t, 270-272
  classification and usage of 270
  effectiveness of 271
  foods with 130t
  legal and ethical aspects of 271
  recommendations for 271-272
  safety of 271
  sports performance factors 270
  theory of 271
vitamin E 97t, 272-274
  classification and usage of 272
  effectiveness of 273
  foods with 130t
  legal and ethical aspects of 273
  recommendations for 273-274
  safety of 273-274
  sports performance factors 272
  theory of 272-273
vitamins, roles of 227t
Vivarin 153
Voy, Robert 109

W

Wadler, Gary 215
weight gain 78
weight loss 78-79
World Championships (1991) 209

Y

yohimbine 97t, 274-275
  classification and usage of 274
  effectiveness of 275
  legal and ethical aspects of 275
  recommendations for 275
  safety of 275
  sports performance factors 274
  theory of 274

Z

zinc 97t, 275-278
  classification and usage of 275
  effectiveness of 276
  foods with 277t
  legal and ethical aspects of 276
  recommendations for 277-278
  safety of 276
  sports performance factors 276
  theory of 276

ABOUT THE AUTHOR

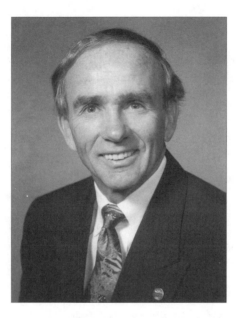

Dr. Mel Williams is a professor in the Department of Exercise Science, Physical Education, and Recreation at Old Dominion University. With more than 30 years of research experience with sports ergogenics, Dr. Williams is both a highly respected scientist and a renowned author. His first book, published in 1974, was one of the first to focus specifically on drugs and sport. His definitive college text, *Nutrition for Fitness and Sport*, is entering its fifth edition. Dr. Williams is a member of the American College of Sports Medicine (ACSM) and the American Alliance for Health, Physical Education, Recreation and Dance (AAHPERD).

Apart from his scientific achievements, Williams has coached football and wrestling at the high school level and cross-country at the college level. A competitive road racer for more than 20 years, his most significant performance came in winning the 50 to 59 age group in the 1989 Boston Marathon.

Dr. Williams lives in Virginia Beach, Virginia. His leisure activities include running and training for road racing, traveling to historic sites, and reading historical novels.

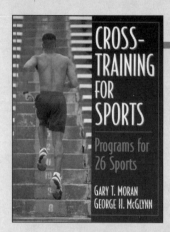
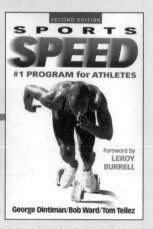
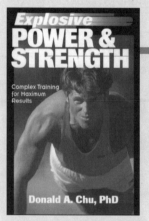